You are What you Eat

DEAR Rajshree

Sue Tai

Tanushree Podder

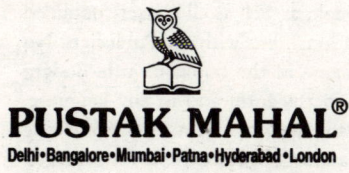

PUSTAK MAHAL®
Delhi•Bangalore•Mumbai•Patna•Hyderabad•London

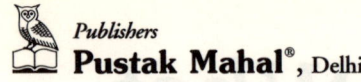

Publishers
Pustak Mahal®, Delhi
J-3/16 , Daryaganj, New Delhi-110002
☎ 23276539, 23272783, 23272784 • *Fax:* 011-23260518
E-mail: info@pustakmahal.com • *Website:* www.pustakmahal.com

London Office
5, Roddell Court, Bath Road, Slough SL3 OQJ, England
E-mail: pustakmahaluk@pustakmahal.com

Sales Centre
10-B, Netaji Subhash Marg, Daryaganj, New Delhi-110002
☎ 23268292, 23268293, 23279900 • *Fax:* 011-23280567
E-mail: rapidexdelhi@indiatimes.com

Branch Offices
Bangalore: ☎ 22234025
E-mail: pmblr@sancharnet.in • pustak@sancharnet.in
Mumbai: ☎ 22010941
E-mail: rapidex@bom5.vsnl.net.in
Patna: ☎ 3294193 • *Telefax:* 0612-2302719
E-mail: rapidexptn@rediffmail.com
Hyderabad: *Telefax:* 040-24737290
E-mail: pustakmahalhyd@yahoo.co.in

© **Pustak Mahal, Delhi**

ISBN 978-81-223-0772-6

Edition : 2007

Printed at : Param Offsetters, Okhla, New Delhi-110020

DEDICATION

This book is dedicated to my beloved husband
who was brave enough to relinquish the demands
of his taste buds in favour of good health

Preface _____

Food is the basic requirement of every living being. But in recent times food has become a very paying business proposition. It is a multi-million dollar industry. While the hotel industry, culinary experts and kitchen queens are raking in money by pampering the taste buds of people; dieticians, doctors and slimming experts are laughing all the way to the bank. The first set is helping the second set of experts in making money. And all this is happening because we have made food the sole purpose of our existence. Instead of eating to live, most of us have started living to eat.

It is difficult to escape the lure of tongue tickling food and lump the food that may not pander to our palate. Not many of us would like to eat boiled chicken or salads if we have the option to indulge in *'Tandoori Murg'* and *'Navratan Korma'*. Nor do we want to trouble our minds with counting calories or balancing them. It is so much more comfortable and hassle-free to let the tongue dictate its terms. In any case, most of us learn to live with the little discomforts caused by unwise eating. It is only when the little discomforts take on giant proportions that we rush to doctors, specialists and dieticians to seek the panacea that will bring relief to our body. First, we spend our hard earned money to buy the discomfort and then spend it again to cure the discomfort.

It may seem ridiculous, but we all end up making the same mistake, most of the time. It isn't as if people are all that ignorant. In these times of spreading awareness it is not likely that many of us are unaware of the ills of the unhealthy diet but we generally lack the will power to put a halt to the consumption of foods that may lead us to disease and discomfort.

Man is a creature of habits. He eats because food has to be eaten at a certain time, whether or not he is hungry. Animals don't do this; they eat only when they are hungry. Our bodies are tuned to signal the need for food but we often ignore the lack of that signal. We take our lunch at a certain time because that happens to be the lunch hour; we have our dinner at a fixed hour because it is dinnertime. Do we ever pause to think if our body requires the food at that time? No, we don't! As a result, our system manifests the excesses in various forms. The indigestion, flatulence, a bloated feeling of discomfort and sluggishness are just a few of those symptoms.

Similarly, we fail to read the signal of our body when it is satiated. Most of us end up eating more food than the body requires. Taste dictates the amount of food that we eat. If the food is very tasty, we overeat and if it is insipid or bland, we take very little of it. And when we overeat, we forget to keep little room for a glass of water.

When I was a little girl of five, I would fuss a lot over my food. I loved eating all kinds of non-vegetarian food and abhorred vegetables and greens, which my mom insisted on feeding me. One day, during dinner when I was creating a big fuss, my father said – "You must remember one simple truth; you are what you eat." At that time, my imagination led me to wonder if I would become a hen if I ate too many eggs, or a pig if I ate too many sausages, both of which I loved! But now I know better.

This simple old saying is a universal truth. We are what we eat. We would naturally be unhealthy if we had unhealthy food habits and healthy if we stuck to eating the healthy and nutritious food, recommended to us by our doctors. It is no great secret that less food never killed anyone but excess does. Excess and the wrong kind of food is the bane of modern society.

It is my earnest hope that the readers of this book will stop for a moment and spare a thought about the kind of food they take, every day, at every meal. There are some golden rules to good health and they are quite easy to follow once a person has made up his mind to remain healthy. Those golden rules have been given in this book, just stick to them and experience the sense of well-being and happiness that comes with following the right diet.

—Tanushree Podder

Contents

Preface ... 7

1. **The Role of Food in Our Body** ... 9
   Food Philosophies ... 10
   Some Macrobiotic Lifestyle Suggestions ... 16
   Change Your Menu as Per the Season ... 19
   The Ayurvedic Philosophy ... 22
   Tibetan Dietary Therapy ... 27
   Traditional Chinese Diet Therapy ... 28
   The Increasing Shift Towards Vegetarianism ... 32
   Healthful Soy ... 35

2. **Foods That Heal** ... 39
   Juice Power ... 48
   Recent Research on Food Power ... 50
   The Healing Power ... 57

3. **Foods That Can Make Us More Intelligent** ... 71
   Memory And The Brain ... 72
   What Are Free Radicals? ... 73
   Memory Food ... 84

4. **Foods That Elevate Our Moods** ... 86
   Dealing with Depression ... 89
   Foods That De-stress ... 91

5. **Unhealthy Food** ... 94
   Food and Allergy ... 121

6. **The Anti-ageing Food Plan** ... 123
   An Anti-ageing secret ... 125
   The 12 Top Anti-ageing Foods ... 130

7. The Yin And Yang of Food ... **135**
    Foods to be Avoided ... 139
    Special Diets ... 140
    Low Triglyceride Diet ... 140
    Low Cholesterol Diet ... 141
    Five Foods for Better Health ... 145
    Five Energy-draining Habits ... 147
    Fruitful Facts ... 148
    Food for Vitality and Vigour ... 154
    Aphrodisiac Foods ... 165
  Table - 1 ... 173
  Table - 2 ... 174
  Table - 3 ... 175

1. The Role of Food in Our Body

Food is the fuel that makes us function, that gives us energy, builds the body and repairs it. Eating is a necessity, but it is also a source of pleasure and a part of our social lives. While in many parts of the world people struggle to eat enough to survive, in affluent countries the culinary delights of food, the domestic routine of mealtimes and other social factors have divorced our eating habits from our real nutritional needs. Hunger, the natural stimulus for eating, has been superseded by habit and custom. The food we eat, far from enhancing our health, is a major contributing factor in serious, widespread health problems, notably heart disease, obesity, cancers, and digestive disorders – the so-called diseases of civilisation. While medical researchers have made definitive recommendations for dietary changes, relatively few of us put their guidelines into practice – at least, until a serious health problem emerges.

The damaging pattern of the modern diet is embedded in social and industrial development – since the turn of the century, greater wealth has led to increased consumption of processed, high-sugar, and high-fat foods, foods that were once regarded as luxuries. There has been a correspondingly sharp decline in the consumption of plain nutritious staples. The general quality has altered too, with modernisation of the food industry involving chemical additives and refining techniques, which have 'denatured' much of the stock in the supermarkets.

Fortunately, the nutritional component in enhancing health and preventing, even curing, illness is now widely recognised. It is well known that a poor diet can exacerbate stress, cause nervous disorders, and affect mental as well as physical development.

There is also increasing concern about food allergies, and the possibility of the potentially toxic cocktail of food additives reacting in the body. Obesity, too, is a matter of widespread anxiety. It is one of the most serious risk factors in many types of diseases and although there is a genetic element, it is largely a result of poor dietary habits. In natural therapies like naturopathy, herbalism and the like, dietary changes play an extremely important part in treating diseases.

Switching to a good diet should not be a matter of making stressful adjustments, such as avoiding all sweet and fatty foods, and living on a monotonous fare of brown rice and vegetables. Fad diets are also not the answer either to ill health or to obesity. They can deprive the body of essential nutrients, and lower the body's metabolic rate. What counts most is establishing a good ratio of nutrients, choosing good quality foods, and being aware of special individual requirements. Within a sensible framework, there is scope for infinite variation, and occasional treats can be enjoyed without harm. You should also combine a balanced diet with a regular exercise programme. But the simplest rule is to choose foods that are as close to their natural state as possible – they are most likely to yield the full range of nutrients that the body needs.

Food Philosophies

There are several kinds of food philosophies that are increasingly finding favour with diet experts. Though ancient in wisdom, they elaborate on the right kind of nutrition to hold the optimum health of mind and body. Most of the popular ones come from Asian countries. The macrobiotic diet and the yogic diet are some of the most scientific theories of food and nutrition. The Ayurvedic food philosophy is also very popular amongst a large segment all over the world. These food philosophies have stood the test of time and are as valid today as they were several centuries ago.

What is Macrobiotics?

The word "macrobiotics" is derived from the Greek words 'Macro' and 'Bios', which means large and life, respectively. A macrobiotic diet is one that helps a person lead a healthy and long life. It is the science that studies the relationship between food and the environment in which we live.

This dietary approach of treatment can be used along with conventional, alternative and other forms of medicine. A macrobiotic diet should include whole grains, beans, fresh vegetables and fruits.

Macrobiotics is a holistic philosophy that aims to achieve balance and peace in people's lives through awareness and common sense living, which includes getting enough rest, eating the way nature intended, being kind and respectful towards oneself and others, and respecting the environment.

Macrobiotics is now popularly known for its success in curing disease, most notably cancer. While a very strict version of the macrobiotic diet can eliminate many cancers, most macrobiotic practitioners recommend a more varied diet based on whole grains, vegetables, beans, and other organic natural foods. By eating the way nature intended, you not only support the ecosystem, but also enhance your own health. To test this yourself, read our seasonal heath tip for easy ways you can transition to natural foods and feel stronger and healthier in the process!

Macrobiotics is based on the Chinese philosophy of yin and yang, the two qualities that balance one another and exist in every natural object and cycle. Yin is the flexible, fluid and feminine side of nature, while yang is the active, alert and masculine part.

Yin qualities are peacefulness, calm, creativity, sociability and a relaxed attitude and behaviour. Most people have a mix of both these qualities. However, when one becomes stronger than the other, a state of imbalance can occur, and result in illness. Too much yin can lead to depression, fatigue and sleeping problems; too much yang can cause tension, irritability, hyperactivity and insomnia.

A macrobiotic therapist would attempt to right that balance by suggesting an increased intake of yin foods for someone suffering from too much yang, and the opposite for someone with too much yin.

A brief history of Macrobiotics

The Macrobiotic Way is a school of thought and action, based upon the use of natural (non-synthetic) materials in our fabrics, our homes and our food. Even many naturally occurring ingredients can be hazardous to our health (e.g. hemlock, opium, sodium, lead); therefore, to determine the correct applications for natural materials, they are classified in accordance with the "Unique Principle".

'The Unique Principle' was introduced to the Western world by George Ohsawa (Yukikazu Sakurazawa), a Japanese businessman, teacher and writer. As a teenager, Ohsawa was diagnosed with tuberculosis by the Japanese doctors and deemed to have little chance of surviving. However, by following the teaching of Sagen Ishizuka, a natural healer who was famous in Japan at the beginning of the 20th century, Ohsawa was able to heal himself. He travelled from Japan to Europe in 1929 and, soon thereafter, began teaching the 'Unique Principle'.

The "Principle", employs the ancient oriental theory of **Yin and Yang** to determine the quality of materials in our universe. Though all aspects of the environment are important in the macrobiotic way of thinking, there is a special emphasis on food. This is because the food we eat becomes our bodies. Therefore, special attention is paid to the quality of that portion of the environment, which we consume. All things, including food, can be classified into a "more yin" or a "more yang" category. Generally speaking, yin (pronounced 'yeen') foods tend to be more sugary and/or watery and/or cold and/or tropical in origin. Yang (pronounced 'yahn') foods tend to be more meaty and/or dry and/or cooked and/or polar, in nature.

Very yang food (e.g. mammal meat, poultry, table salt, ginseng), as well as very yin food (e.g. sugar, euphoric drugs, strong alcoholic beverages) are generally avoided. These foods are often called "extreme foods". Balanced foods, which are not so "extreme", compose the standard macrobiotic diet. Cereal grains reside at the balance between yin and yang, but even they are involved in the yin and yang classification (everything has yin and yang components; nothing is "neutral"). Therefore, whole grains and their derivatives (pasta, bread, hominy) are considered the mainstay of the diet. All ancient civilisations had used a grain-based element as the main diet.

Along with whole grain, the diet is comprised of bean and bean products, a wide variety of vegetables, kelp and other sea vegetables, many excellent soups and condiments, nuts and occasional fish and fruit. Macrobiotic people pay close attention to their personal condition and they adjust the yin and yang quality of their diets, as required to maintain a healthy life and happiness. In addition to classification by type, the quality of the food is also considered. Vegetables should be organically grown.

Fish and sea vegetables should be harvested from deep, clean water or from coastal areas located far from city and industrial pollution. Also, genetically engineered foods, even grains and beans, are to be avoided. Organic food grown from traditional, open-pollinated seed is best. To some individuals, this entire process may sound unlikely or farfetched. In that case, it is important to know that the macrobiotic diet has healed thousands of individuals; some, from very life threatening illnesses, such as cancer and heart disease and even enabled diabetics to wean themselves away from insulin. There are many well-documented case histories of people who have healed themselves through macrobiotic procedures.

Macrobiotics is used to improve health, thinking, sharpen the senses and elevate consciousness. It utilises the same fundamentals as Feng Shui (composition in space) and 9 Ki (composition in time). But in this case, these basic principles are applied directly to our physical bodies and our lives.

General dietary and lifestyle guidelines are not intended to define a specific regimen that one must follow, as additional adjustments are required for individual application, which vary according to personal situations.

Macrobiotic dietary suggestions

For occasional use:
- Fish and Seafood
- Seasonal Fruits
- Nuts, Seeds, and Other Natural Snacks

Food suggestions for persons living in a temperate climate

Whole cereal grains:
- 50% by weight
- Organically grown, whole grain is recommended, which can be cooked in a variety of cooking methods.

- Grains include: Brown rice, barley, millet, oats, corn, rye, wheat, and buckwheat. While whole grains are recommended, a small portion of the recommended percentage of grains may consist of noodles or pasta, unyeasted whole grain breads, and other partially processed whole cereal grains.

Vegetables

- Approximately 20 - 30% by weight
- Local and organically grown vegetables are recommended, with the majority being cooked in various styles such as lightly steamed or boiled, sautéed with a small amount of unrefined, cold pressed oil. A small portion may be used as fresh salad, and a very small volume as pickles.
- Vegetables for daily use include: green cabbage, kale, broccoli, cauliflower, collards, pumpkin, watercress, parsley, Chinese cabbage, bok choy, dandelion, mustard greens, daikon greens, scallion, onions, daikon radish, turnips, burdock, carrots, winter squash such as butternut, buttercup, and acorn squash.
- For occasional use in season (2 to 3 times a week); cucumber, celery, lettuce, herbs such as dill, chives.
- Vegetables not recommended for regular use include: eggplant, peppers, spinach, beets, and zucchini.

Beans and Sea Vegetables

- Approximately 5 - 10 % by weight
- The most suitable beans for regular use are azuki beans, chickpeas, and lentils. Other beans may be used on occasion. Bean products such as tofu, tempeh, and natto can also be used. Sea vegetables such as nori, wakame, kombu, hiziki, arame, dulse, and agar-agar are an important part of the macrobiotic diet as they provide important vitamins and minerals.

Soups

- Approximately 5 - 10 % by weight
- Soups may be made with vegetables, sea vegetables, grains, or beans. Seasonings include miso, tamari soy sauce, and sea salt.

Beverages

Recommended beverages include:

- Roasted bancha twig tea, stem tea, roasted brown rice tea, roasted barley tea, dandelion root tea, and cereal grain coffee. Any traditional tea that does not have an aromatic fragrance or a stimulating effect can also be used.
- When drinking water, spring or good quality well water is recommended, without ice.

Occasional Foods

- Fish, 1 - 3 times per week approximately 5 - 10 % by weight of that day's consumption. Recommended fish include fresh white-meat fish such as flounder, sole, cod, carp, halibut or trout.
- Fruit or fruit desserts, made from fresh or dried fruit, may be served two or three times a week. Local and organically grown fruits are preferred. If you live in a temperate climate, avoid tropical and semi-tropical fruit and instead, eat temperate climate fruits such as apples, pears, plums, peaches, apricots, berries and melons. Frequent use of fruit juice is not advisable.
- Lightly roasted nuts and seeds such as pumpkin, sesame, and sunflower seeds. Peanuts, walnuts and pecans may be enjoyed as an occasional snack.
- Rice syrup, barley malt, amasake, and mirin may be used as sweeteners.
- Brown rice vinegar or umeboshi vinegar may be used occasionally for a sour taste.

Recommended Condiments

- Gomashio, seaweed powder (kelp, kombu, wakame, and other sea vegetables), Sesame seaweed powder, umeboshi plums, tekka, pickles and sauerkraut made using sea salt, miso, or tamari.

Additional Dietary Suggestions

- Only vegetable oil should be used for cooking. To improve your health, it is preferable to use only unrefined sesame or corn oil in moderate amounts.

- Salt should be naturally processed sea salt. Traditional, non-chemicalised shoyu or tamari soy sauce and miso may also be used as seasonings.

Foods to Eliminate

- Meat, animal proteins, dairy products and eggs (including butter, yoghurt, ice cream, milk and cheese), refined sugars, chocolate, molasses, honey, other simple sugars and foods treated with them, and vanilla.
- Tropical or semi-tropical fruits and fruit juices, soda, artificial drinks and beverages, coffee, coloured tea, and all aromatic stimulating teas such as mint or peppermint tea.
- All artificially coloured, preserved, sprayed, or chemically treated foods. All refined and polished grains, flours, and their derivatives; mass-produced industrialized food including all canned, frozen, and irradiated foods.
- Hot spices, any aromatic stimulating food or food accessory, artificial vinegar, and strong alcoholic beverages.

Macrobiotics also recommend

- Increasing the quantity of complex carbohydrates
- Decreasing the intake of salt
- A total taboo on junk food

Note — Since these dietary rules are of Chinese origin, some of the elements may not be locally available. For such elements, substitutes can be used.

Some Macrobiotic Lifestyle Suggestions

In order to establish a firm foundation of natural health, physiological stability, and adaptability, it is vital that the following factors in our daily lives that have led to symptoms or suffering or sickness are recognised, so that we may seek or correct them. Macrobiotics is believed to be the natural cycle of life, an example of the universal rhythms of yin and yang, which occur everywhere and in everything. Macrobiotic practitioners urge you to live each day happily, without being pre-occupied with your condition, or dwelling on negative thoughts, ideas or emotions.

It is a fundamental belief that nature is essential to life, and that regular contact with nature is necessary to enjoy optimum health and well-being. There are some daily practices, which are helpful in creating a more stable and harmonious lifestyle.

- Eat only when hungry.
- Proper chewing is important for good digestion and assimilation of nutrients.
- Eat in an orderly and relaxed manner. When you eat, sit in a good posture and take a moment to express gratitude for the food.
- You may eat regularly two or three times per day, as much as you want, provided the proportion is generally correct and each mouthful is thoroughly chewed. It is best to leave the table satisfied but not full.
- Drink liquids moderately, only when thirsty.
- For the deepest and most restful sleep, retire before midnight and avoid eating at least 2 to 3 hours before sleeping.
- Bathe as needed but try to avoid lengthy hot baths or showers, as they can deplete the body of minerals and have a weakening effect. Preferably, take brief baths or showers with a moderate temperature. If you feel fatigued after bathing you may drink a small cup of shoyubancha, or miso soup to replenish your energy.
- Use cosmetics and cleaning products that are made from natural, non-toxic ingredients. Avoid chemically perfumed products. For care of the teeth, brush with natural preparations. To maintain healthy skin function, which plays a vital part in the excretory system's regular discharging of toxins, avoid using chemically produced cosmetics and body care products. Try to use natural cosmetics from vegetable sources only.
- As much as possible, wear cotton clothing, especially for under-garments. Avoid wearing synthetic or woollen clothing directly on the skin. Avoid wearing excessive accessories on the fingers, wrists, neck, or any other part of the body.
- Spend time outdoors if strength permits. Walk on the grass, beach or soil up to half-hour every day. Spend some time in direct sunlight. Get plenty of fresh air, and when you can, walk barefoot on the soil, grass or beach. Keep large green plants in your home to increase the circulation of fresh oxygen, and open windows wherever possible. It is best to

use central heating and air-conditioning only to the extent necessary for reasonable comfort. Allow yourself to experience the natural seasonal changes of temperature appropriate to the climate where you live.

- Exercise regularly. Activities may include walking, yoga, martial arts, dance, etc.
- Keep your home in good order, especially the areas where food is prepared and served.
- To revitalise the blood and stimulate circulation, scrub and massage the whole body with a hot, damp cotton towel or flannel until your skin becomes flushed, each morning or night. At least scrub the arms, legs, hands and feet, including each finger and toe.
- Avoid using electric cooking devices such as ovens and cooking ranges or microwave oven. The use of a gas or wood stove is preferred.
- Use earthenware, cast iron, or stainless steel cookware rather than aluminium or Teflon-coated pots.
- Minimize the frequent use of television and computer display units. When using a computer, protect yourself from potentially harmful electromagnetic fields with a protective shield over the screen and other safety devices.
- Greet everyone happily and with appreciation.
- Initiate and maintain a regular correspondence with all family members, expressing thanks for their part in your life.
- Enlarge your circle of friends and acquaintances, including people from different lifestyles.
- Share your food more often by having people around; food prepared in large quantities is more satisfying and the act of sharing food is a universal gesture of human kindness and brotherhood.
- Put aside some time each day for peace and quiet, and thank your forebears and teachers for their help. Repeat your dedication to aid and support those who look to you for guidance.

Effects of change in diet

Sometimes a sudden change in the dietary pattern may cause certain problems. However, once the body gets used to the new pattern everything would be normal. This occurs due to elimination of accumulated toxins from the system. These problems, however, differ depending on the body constitution.

Some of the common symptoms are:
- Aches and pains
- Fatigue
- Chills
- Sweating
- Frequent urination
- Body odour
- Constipation
- Irregular or temporary cessation of menstruation
- Insomnia

Change your Menu as per the Season

Follow some of these principles and you will very soon feel the difference. There have been many cases where cancer and diabetes patients have adopted this diet pattern and highly benefited from it.

What is a Healthy Diet?

A healthy diet is one in which the food you eat contains all the nutrients needed by the body for it to grow, heal and function normally on a day-to-day basis. A balanced diet provides energy, and allows you to function at your optimum level, free from disease and malaise.

There are three essential nutrient food groups – proteins, carbohydrates and fats plus minerals and vitamins. You also need water, which is found in most foods and makes up a large proportion of our body. Roughly speaking, proteins should make up about 15% of the diet, carbohydrates 60% or more and fats a maximum of 25-30%. Vitamins and minerals are found within each of these groups, and a balanced diet should have all or most represented in adequate levels. Dietary fibre is also very important.

Surveys show that most macrobiotic practitioners use the diet as a basis for healthy living but also enjoy a 5-10% intake of other foods either socially, or to give a dietary balance. Emphasis is placed on the art of cooking, and on the variety of cooking styles and ingredients.

Foods to be excluded from the diet include sugar, spices and alcohol (said to be too much yin), and meat, eggs and cheese (too much yang). These foods are generally believed to be too strong for human consumption, unbalancing the system and causing illness. The best-balanced foods containing yin and yang are –

- Yin – fruit, leafy green vegetables, nuts and seeds, tofu and tempeh, fruit and vegetable juices, jams (made without refined sugar), barley malt.
- Yang – wholegrain cereals, such as brown rice, bread, flour, whole oats, root vegetables such as potatoes, parsnips and turnips, fish and shellfish, cottage cheese, beans, peas and lentils, salt, miso and shoyu soya sauce.

The Macrobiotic Logic

Practitioners believe that macrobiotics changes the condition of your blood, which is made of three main components – plasma, red blood cells and white blood cells. Plasma amounts to about 50% of the cells, and changes every ten days. Therefore, changes in your health will be noticeable in ten-day cycles.

When you begin a macrobiotic programme, you will notice some large changes during the first ten days, mainly as a reaction or a 'discharge process'. Tiredness, irritability, sweating, insomnia and cravings are common. After about 10-30 days, people generally tend to feel brighter, and more alert, with an increased appetite, and a calmer, more focused and flexible outlook.

When people continue for 6-8 months on a macrobiotic programme, their blood will show a great improvement and have perfectly balanced yin and yang. If regular physical activity is kept up, and there is plenty of variety in the diet and lifestyle, then chronic ailments should normally show noticeable improvement.

Changing your diet is a very big step approaching it in the right way and getting support and feedback is essential to minimise mistakes. It takes commitment and patience to practise, but practitioners say that when it becomes effortless and you genuinely enjoy the food you eat, you have become macrobiotic.

The following principles are recommended for people who live in temperate zones:

1. Each meal should be based on vegetable products with occasional supplements of animal food, if necessary.
2. Whole cereal grains should constitute more than half of the meal, with occasional supplements of beans.
3. Most vegetable should be cooked rather than raw and chosen for seasonal variation. Locally grown produce is preferable to that grown at a distance and therefore out of season.
4. Sea vegetables may be used as a supplement.
5. Fruits and nuts grown in the same climate may also be used.
6. Animal food should comprise less than 15% of the meal and should always be eaten with vegetables.
7. Food should be mainly seasoned with unrefined sea salt and vegetable oil.

The Problem of Acid and Alkaline

Determining the right combination of acid and alkaline foods to produce a healthy balance in the blood may sometimes be confusing, but if we think in terms of yin and yang we soon learn to distinguish between the two food groups.

As a rule of thumb, vegetable species are generally more yin while animal foods tend to be yang. There are, however, different degrees of these two qualities. For example, vegetables with more yin qualities cool the body in hot weather and produce physical and mental expansion while yang quality cooked vegetables activate the metabolism and increase body temperature. In general practice, if we use animal products it is advisable to choose yin quality vegetable to harmonize and balance the meal.

Two examples to demonstrate different properties of vegetables:
- Celery grows in a warm climate, is long in shape, fragile and watery, has a strong smell and taste and is pale green in colour. Celery therefore has many yin properties.
- Carrots, on the other hand, are more compact, grow slowly in a cool climate, are orange in colour and mild in taste and

21

take longer cooking time. Although a vegetable, it is more yang in character than celery.

The Ayurvedic Philosophy

According to ayurveda, there are positive and negative attributes of diet. Since ayurveda deals with a holistic approach to healing, it covers the diet factor in depth.

Ayurveda has categorised personality traits into three different kinds, based on the food we eat – the *Satvic* or spiritual quality, *Rajasic* or active quality, and *Tamasic* or material quality of the mind are all affected by the food we eat. The activating *Rajasic* quality may dominate or combine with the other two qualities to form different mental tendencies in man; spiritually active, intellectually active, or materially active.

Satvic food is one that can be digested easily and brings balance to one's mind. It helps in building immunity and improving the healing response in those who are unwell. *Satvic* food is all food closest to the natural form and includes milk, milk products, fruits, most fresh vegetables except garlic, onion, scallions, and chives.

Whole grain cereals like most lentils, sprouts and natural sweeteners like jaggery, honey are also included in *Satvic* diet. Also included in this category are the natural oils like ghee, butter and vegetable oils.

Satvic food is moderately cooked with few spices and less fat. Chillies and black pepper are not used in cooking. Common spices like turmeric, ginger, cinnamon, coriander, aniseed and cardamom are, however, used in *Satvic* cooking. Eating raw foods is not considered *Satvic* as they harbour a lot of parasites and microbes. According to ayurveda, raw foods are known to weaken the digestive system and reduce *ojas* which is synonymous with vital energy also known as *prana*. Prana is also known as 'Chi' (and 'Qi') or 'jing'. Simplified, it means the life force.

The proper functioning of the mind and spiritual development depend on ojas. A person who follows the Satvic food habits is known to possess a clear mind, is balanced, moderate in habits and focussed. He usually avoids intoxicants like alcohol, stimulants like

22

tea, coffee, tobacco and non-vegetarian food. A Satvic person is also supposed to be spiritually aware.

Rajasic food is one that is fresh but heavy to digest. Those who indulge in heavy physical activity should eat such food. It includes non-vegetarian food like meat, fish, eggs, chicken, all whole pulses and dals, which are not sprouted. Foods prepared from sour, salty, spicy 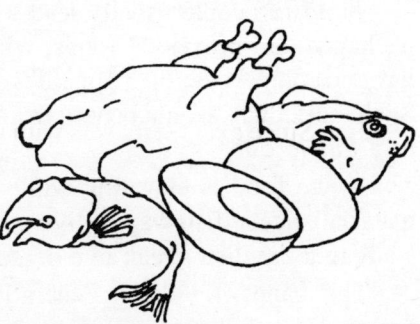 ingredients increase Rajasic qualities. Hot spices like chillies, pepper, vegetables, including onions and garlic, are all included under this category.

Rajasic food is cooked fresh and is of high quality and nutrient density. It also contains more spices and oil than *Satvic* cooking.

This kind of food is known to make a person long for sensual stimulation. He is usually aggressive in nature in a positive way and is of energetic disposition. He is interested in power, prestige, position and prosperity. But he is in control of his life and not obsessed by the power and position. A *Rajasic* personality loves to enjoy life.

Tamasic food includes all kinds that are not fresh and are unnatural, overcooked, stale and processed. All foods made from refined flour, pastries, pizzas, burgers, chocolates, soft drinks, stimulants like tea, coffee, tobacco, intoxicants like alcohol and wines fall under the *Tamasic* category. Even canned and preserved foods like jams, jellies, pickles and fermented food come under this group. Fried foods, sweets made from sugar, ice creams, pudding and most modern day junk foods, spicy, salty, sweet, and fatty foods are also included in this list.

Tamas means darkness, implying stagnation in a person and degeneration in health. The *tamasic* personality suffers from intense mood swings, insecurities, desires, cravings and is unable to deal with others in a balanced manner. They have little regard for the welfare of others and tend to be very self-centred. Their nervous systems and heart do not function optimally, such individuals age very fast and usually suffer from degenerative conditions like cancer, heart disease, diabetes, arthritis, chronic fatigue etc.

Tamasic people usually lead a sedentary lifestyle and enjoy packaged and processed foods, which are rich in calories. They have no control over their appetites and indulge in mindless eating. Such individuals would benefit from switching from a *tamasic* diet to a *Satvic* one.

Satvic food is elevating while *Rajasic* foods lead man to a materialistic, selfish way of living. Worst is *Tamasic* food, which leads to a devilish streak in a person.

The bane of today's generation is that they are *Tamasic* personalities. Self-centred, insecure and ailing, they are reaching a point of no return. The very food that has become an epitome of fashion is of unhealthy nature. We are leaving the wisdom of *Satvic* food and rushing towards the ills of an unhealthy *tamasic* diet. No wonder our society is degenerating into a violent, self-seeking, power hungry and uncaring one.

The Six 'Rasas' (tastes)

According to ayurveda, there are six types of tastes and each taste has a different effect on digestion. Taste also has a long-term or post digestive effect on the body and its metabolism (*vipaaka*). A *rasa* can be light or heavy, moist or dry. Light tastes are easier to digest and assimilate, while those that are heavy require more energy to digest

1. *Tikta rasa* is bitter taste. In many regions of the country, bitter preparation is served at the beginning of a meal because it activates and speeds up digestion. When the body becomes toxic, hot or itchy, *tikta rasa* is the best corrective measure. However, care should be taken that excessive bitter taste is not included in the diet as it can lead to problems like loss of appetite, weight loss, dry skin or headaches.

2. *Amla rasa* or sour taste stimulates appetite and adds taste to food. It helps to expel gas and combat anorexia. Sour taste can act as an anti-coagulant also. Excess of sour taste can, however, aggravate thirst and cause burning sensation in the throat and chest. Sharp qualities of mind such as witticism and intellect are increased by sour foods but excess can lead to anaemia, haemorrhage, vertigo and vision problems.

3. *Madhura rasa* or sweet taste is popular amongst most people. Any food that is nourishing and satisfying has a sweet taste. Eating foods with *madhura rasa* is known to elevate heaviness, coldness and physical energy. Sweet foods are useful in easing bowel movement and also have a diuretic effect apart from calming the brain. However, an excess can lead to lethargy, emotional dependency, obesity, loss of appetite, diabetes, swelling of lymph, nodes etc.

4. *Lavana rasa* or salty taste adds relish to food and activates the flow of saliva and gastric juices. Excessive salt intake can create weight gain, heaviness, grey hair, premature wrinkling, hair fall, skin diseases and gastric disorders. In ayurveda it is also believed to lead to cravings and uncontrollable desires.

5. *Katu rasa* or pungent taste relates to hot and spicy food. It causes a burning sensation and heating and drying effect, which results in thirst. Pungent taste stimulates the body and makes body fluids like sweat, tears, saliva, mucus and blood flow freely. So digestion increases and congested tissues are cleaned out. However, excess pungency can result in swollen lips, burning skin, thirst and dizziness.

6. *Kashaaya rasa* or astringent taste is not an easy one to define. It is light and sedative and causes granulation, absorption and stiffness. *Kashaaya rasa* is cooling and constrictive. It stops the flow of secretions such as sweat and tears. It controls anxiety and excitement. An excessive inclusion of astringent tasting foods in the diet may lead to constipation and dryness of the mouth along with abdominal bloating.

According to ayurveda, it is advisable to include foods that contain all the six *rasas* in the meal because they control our well-being and create dietary balance. Excessive consumption of any of these could result in adverse effects.

The Acid and Alkali Balance

It is essential to balance the acid and alkali levels in our bodily systems. This fact has been known to ancient healers and ayurveda lays down many rules to balance these two factors. The pH factor indicates the acidity and alkalinity of the body and plays a vital role in body chemistry. Normal pH value is 7 and any value under this indicates acidity, while values above 7 are an indication of alkalinity.

The pH value of saliva and urine is 6 and 6.8 respectively which shows that they are slightly acidic in nature. These are the average values; any value above this would indicate and alkaline nature, while anything lower would indicate a more acidic nature. High acidic levels in the body can cause several problems like acidity, heart-burn, indigestion, headaches, nervous disorders, excessive hunger and even drowsiness.

Acidosis causes many diseases like high blood pressure, skin diseases, frequent cough, cold and fever, rheumatism, premature ageing and low immunity. Considering these, one would think that alkalinity is better but one can't be further from the truth because a high level of alkalinity in the body causes sluggishness, lethargy, water retention, lack of concentration, lack of drive and will power etc. However, studies indicate that people with higher alkaline levels are less prone to diseases and have a stronger immune system.

Acidosis can easily be controlled through a carefully monitored diet. All flesh foods, refined foods like sugars and maida, coffee, grains like wheat, oats, barley etc, pulses and eggs are high in acid content. On the other hand, foods like leafy vegetables, fruits, mushrooms etc are alkaline in nature. Citrus fruits, though acidic in taste, become alkaline when digested and help in restoring the balance of acid and alkali in the body. Foods that contain higher levels of calcium, magnesium, potassium and sodium reduce acidity and help in maintaining the alkalinity level.

To balance the acid and alkali levels, 80% of the food that we consume should be alkaline, while 20% should be acidic. This means that we should incorporate more of root vegetables like yam, beetroot, carrots, radish etc in the menu, while avoiding acid forming foods such as wheat, oat, rice, barley, bread, fish, eggs, pulses etc. Most green vegetables like peas, cucumber, gourds, lady finger, cabbages, onions, beans, cauliflower etc, are also alkaline in nature. Adding fruit juices is a very safe method of adding alkali to the body. Fruit and vegetable juices are extremely beneficial for health.

Leafy green vegetables like spinach, methi, beet greens, spring onion leaves, radish leaves, amaranth leaves are particularly useful while trying to balance the acid-alkali levels and it is advisable to include them in plentiful.

Tibetan Dietary Therapy

As in Chinese medicine, the most fundamental type of treatment in Tibetan medicine is the modification of behaviour and diet.

Tibetan medicine is a "nomadic" type of medicine, that is, since the doctor travelled around the country on a yak to treat patients, he was only able to come around once every six months to a year. So not only was dietary regulation a less intrusive form of treatment, but the patient could also adhere to these instructions without constant supervision from the doctor.

According to Tibetan medicine, inadequate, excessive, or inappropriate diet will result in disease. Inadequate would be considered not enough quantity of food and liquids to sustain one, i.e. undereating or inappropriate fasting or not having enough of the proper foods. Excessive means eating too much at one time or over the course of the day. Intake of food while there is still an undigested meal present will lead to problems. Buddha stated that stagnant food (in the stomach) is the original cause of most disease.

To avoid stagnant food, it is recommended that the stomach only be filled to ¾ full. One half should be food and one-quarter liquid. Inappropriate diet is one in which unwholesome foods, foods that one is not accustomed to or are not appropriate to one's ailments are eaten. It also includes the practice of untimely dining. Unwholesome foods are those that are not fresh, or whole foods. This includes any "junk foods" and highly processed foods. Untimely dining refers to eating the wrong foods during a particular season.

Normal Diet

Food types in Tibetan medicine are classified as grain, meat, oil, vegetables (cooked), prepared foods (congee, cooked rice, soups, stew) and liquids.

Grain: two types – without pods and with pods.

Non-podded: rice, millet and barley.

Podded: beans.

Meat: flesh of land animals and fowl.

Oils: butter, grain oils, marrow and fats.

Vegetables: assorted, cooked.

Liquids: milk, water, beer, and others.

Traditional Chinese Diet Therapy

Guided by fundamental theories of Traditional Chinese Medicine, Traditional Chinese Diet (TCD) therapy is concerned with the study of how to make good use of foods and natural nutriments, as well as the Chinese *materia medica* to preserve health, prevent and heal diseases, quicken their recovery, and slow down ageing. TCD has remained an important component of traditional Chinese medicine, the same as acupuncture, herbology, Tui Na (massage), Qi Gong, etc. The therapeutic effect of TCD has been proven through the clinical practice of centuries, especially in areas like preventive medicine, rehabilitation and gerontology.

TCD is based on the fundamentals of traditional Chinese medicine in the aspects of both theory and clinical practice, i.e. the theory of Yin-Yang, Five Elements, Zang-Fu organs, meridians, etiology and pathogenesis, diagnostic methods, therapeutic principles, etc.

TCD concentrates on the idea of holistic entity and the principle of curing diseases in accordance with the differential diagnosis of syndromes. It is believed in Traditional Chinese Medicine that foods as well as herbs have different natures and flavours, accounting for their actions of reinforcing or reducing bodily benefits.

Foods are able to balance Yin and Yang, and Qi and blood in the body. To prevent and cure diseases, both foods and medicines could exert important roles since they share the same source, are based on the same theory, and have similar medicinal actions. Hence, food and herbs are combined in clinical use.

The Four Natures

Foods, the same as herbs, could also be classified into "four natures" i.e. "cold", "hot", "warm" and "cool" in line with their actions and curative effects. The foods of "cold" or "cool" property can be used to treat hot-natured diseases, while "hot" or "warm" foods are used in treating cold-natured diseases. Some foods may be neutral in nature.

Foods cold or cool in nature: Barley, millet, buckwheat, green bean, coix seed, celery, spinach, lettuce, green cabbage stems, turnips (white), bamboo shoot, lily bulb, lotus root, eggplant, tomato, water melon, white gourd, sponge gourd, cucumber, bitter melon, apple, pear, orange, banana, rabbit's meat, duck's meat, duck's egg, crab, fresh water snail, kelp, laver, green tea, soy sauce, table salt, rock candy.

Foods hot or warm in nature: Glutinous rice, Chinese sorghum, pumpkin, hot pepper, ginger, scallion, onion, leek, funnel green, garlic, parsley, mustard greens, dates, walnut kernel, plum, arbutus, pomegranate, longan, peach, cherry, apricot, chestnut, pineapple, spirit, vinegar, black tea, pepper, coffee, chicken, turkey, mutton, venison, spotted silver carp, grass fish, trout, red sugar.

Foods neutral in nature: Polished rice, wheat, corn, soybean, pea, small red bean, cabbage, cauliflower, carrot, fungus, silver fungus, mushroom, yam, day-lily buds, peanut, potato, lemon, grapes, cherry apple, olive, lotus seed, pork, beef, spring chicken, pigeon's meat, quail's meat, egg, carp, mandarin fish, eel, turtle, jelly fish, abalone, white sugar, honey, jasmine tea, wulong tea.

The Five Flavours

The five flavours refer to the concept of five kinds of taste of foods or drugs, i.e., pungent, sweet, sour, bitter and salty.

1. *Pungent flavour:* Ginger, scallion, garlic, hot pepper, pepper, cayenne pepper, onion, leek, spirit.

2. *Sweet flavour:* Potato, lotus root, wheat, polished rice, pea, milk, pork, chestnut, date, honey.

3. *Sour flavour:* Tomato, tangerine, plum, lemon, grape, papaya, haw, cherry apple, pomegranate, and vinegar.

4. *Bitter flavour:* Bitter melon, almond, lily bulb, orange peel, tea, coffee, bitter green, arrowroot, pig liver.

5. *Salty flavour:* Barley, millet, dried purple sea weed, kelp, jelly fish, pork, beef, crab, table salt.

In traditional Chinese medicine, the concept of 'flavour' is not limited to tastes, but also covers the actions of foods e.g. licorice is sweet in flavour, but it can also be used to tone Qi, ease cramp and harmonize other materials. It has been acknowledged in traditional Chinese medicine that herbs or foods may exert different effects because of the specific flavour of each kind. Pungent flavour tends to disperse (e.g. opening the pores of the skin and causing perspiration); sourness gathers (astringent effect); bitter flavour removes pathological heat; and salty flavour softens hard masses. In clinical practice or everyday life, it is often noticed that: such pungent foods as ginger and scallion are used to treat common cold; sweet-flavoured foods such as chestnut and jujube can be used to treat weakness and deficiency; lemon and black plum of sour flavour can be used to stop diarrhoea; bitter melons, bitter greens of bitter flavour are helpful in the treatment of febrile diseases.

Meridian Tropism

Meridian tropism is about the body parts herbs or foods act on since they have strong affinity to internal organs and meridians.

1. Some foods tropistic to Heart meridian: Wheat, lotus seeds, lily bulb, red bean, longan, and pork skin.
2. Some foods tropistic to Liver meridian: Tomato, sponge gourd, papaya, haw, eel, pork liver.
3. Some foods tropistic to Spleen meridian: Polished rice, wheat, millet, snap bean, watermelon, and pork.
4. Some foods tropistic to Lung meridian: Ginger, onion, (white) turnip, pear, lily bulb, almond, water chestnut.
5. Some foods tropistic to Kidney meridian: Duck's meat, mutton, walnut kernel, sesame, prawn.

Attribution of Five Flavours

In terms of the theory of five flavour it is held in traditional Chinese medicine that bitter attributes to the heart, sour to the liver, sweet to the spleen, pungent to the lungs and salty to the kidneys.

Congeneric Theory

This theory is related also to the meridian tropism, i.e. treating disorders of human body with certain internal organs or tissues of animals. For instance, animal liver (or heart, or thyroid gland, or reproductive organs) can be used to treat liver (or heart or thyroid gland or sexual function) disorders.

(Even nowadays, this theory is still applicable in modern medicine, e.g. the use of insulin to treat diabetes and thyroid hormone to treat hyperthyroidism.)

Digestion Facts

Do you know it takes about 13 hours to digest raw vegetables, fruits and sprouts, while cooked vegetables and pulses take about 24 hours before the system is able to absorb the nutrients? As for non-vegetarian and fried stuff, it takes up to 72 hours before it can break the nutrients into an absorbable form.

That explains the extra long intestine inside our belly. Our small intestine measures about 22 feet (7 metres) and the large intestine is about 5 feet (1.5 metres) long. Together they measure about 27 feet (8.5 metres).

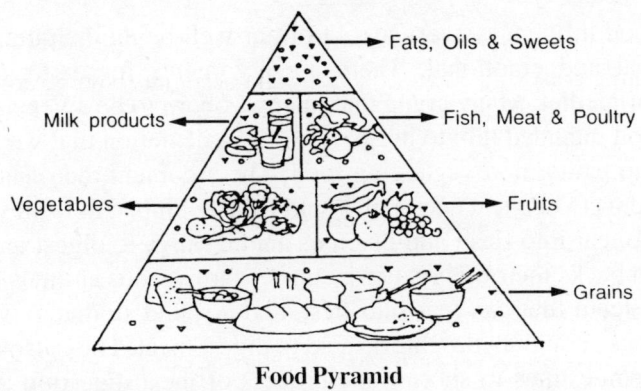

Fats, Oils & Sweets

Milk products

Fish, Meat & Poultry

Vegetables

Fruits

Grains

Food Pyramid

Effect of Food on the Mind

Proper foods in the right combinations are necessary for sustenance of the body; they also exert a definite influence upon the mind. Everything we eat produces a sensation on the palate as well as certain chemical effects on the body and brain. The sensations created by the food determine a specific mentality. Meat eating produces gross material reactions that develop the material or animal mental tendencies, whereas eating raw fruits and vegetables helps to reinforce and develop the spiritual qualities.

The Increasing Shift Towards Vegetarianism

"Those who eat flesh are but eating grains and vegetables secondhand..... How much better to get it direct, by eating the food that God provided for our use!"   **– Ellen G. White**

Vegetarians do not eat meat for health, philosophical or moral reasons. Some, such as Jains and Brahmins, are vegetarians because of religious beliefs.

There are three main types of vegetarians: lacto-ovo-vegetarians, who eat dairy foods and eggs; lacto-vegetarians, who eat dairy foods, but no eggs; and vegans who consume no animal foods of any type.

Food influences every aspect of our well-being including the physical and emotional. There are arguments for and against vegetarian diet. Many argue that man was born to be a vegetarian and God intended him to be so; it is only a deviation that we have taken to eating non-vegetarian food. The argument that if nature wanted us to be meat eaters, it would have equipped us with sharp teeth to tear into flesh and given us acidic saliva to digest animal protein backs their theory. For instance, carnivorous animals have claws, teeth that can tear into flesh and a round stomach, which produces enough hydrochloric acid to digest meat. They also have shorter intestines to shorten the process of meat digestion and a liver that is equipped to get rid of excess uric acid.

That man was created as a vegetarian is borne out by the molars that are designed to crush and grind. Our saliva is alkaline in nature, which is perfect to digest plant protein; we have a stomach and greater length of intestines, designed for vegetarian food. The liver of human beings is also not equipped get rid of excess uric acid that the animal protein breakdown produces. That is one of the prime reasons for the painful disease called gout.

On the other hand the proponents of non-vegetarianism argue that all food that can be digested by man should be considered normal and healthy. Their point is that only non-vegetarian food can provide all the elements of a nutritious diet and so it is healthier than the vegan diet.

There are many factors against the consumption of meat. Animal protein is tough to digest and the food putrefies inside the system creating toxins that are harmful to the body.

Benefits of Vegetarianism

Vegetarian diets are typically lower than non-vegetarian diets in total fat, saturated fat, and cholesterol. These factors are associated with increased risk of obesity, coronary heart disease, high blood pressure, diabetes mellitus, and some forms of cancer. Thus, it is logical that vegetarian diets are healthy and nutritionally adequate when appropriately planned.

Vegetarians have lower average blood cholesterol and therefore a reduced risk of coronary artery disease. They have a lower risk of obesity and suffer from fewer digestive problems compared to non-vegetarians.

Plant foods have been shown to have "chemo-preventive" properties. Risk of lung cancer in heavy smokers has been shown to be reduced in populations eating generous amounts of plant foods, and risk of breast, prostate and other cancers is substantially lower in populations that consume vegetarian diets.

Researchers have identified eight food groups, each of which has unique cancer-preventing qualities. All eight groups come from the plant kingdom. Conversely, animal product consumption is implicated in a host of degenerative diseases including cancer and heart disease, and animal-source foods in general provide little or no protection against most health conditions other than starvation.

Nutrients to Consider in a Vegetarian Diet

Protein: You don't need to eat animal products to have enough protein in your diet. Plant proteins alone can provide enough of the essential and non-essential amino acids, as long as sources of dietary protein are varied and caloric intake is high enough to meet energy needs. Whole grains, legumes, vegetables, seeds and nuts all contain both essential and non-essential amino

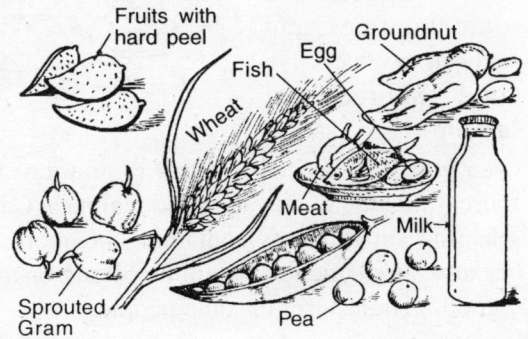

Fruits with hard peel • Fish • Wheat • Egg • Groundnut • Meat • Milk • Sprouted Gram • Pea

acids. Soy protein has been shown to be equal to proteins of animal origin.

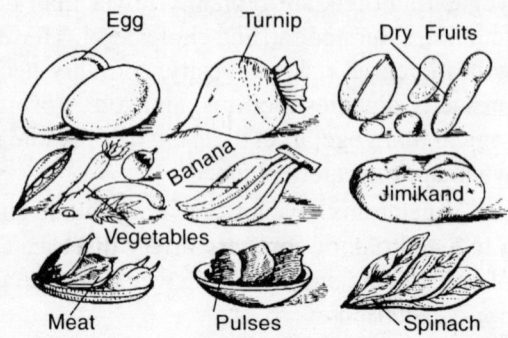

Iron: Vegetarians may have a greater risk of iron deficiency than non-vegetarians. The richest sources of iron are red meat, liver and egg yolk – all high in cholesterol. Dried beans, spinach, enriched products; brewer's yeast and dried fruits are all good plant sources of iron.

Vitamin B-12: Comes naturally from animal sources only. Vegans need a reliable source of vitamin B-12, which can be found in some fortified (not enriched) breakfast cereals, fortified soy beverages, some brands of nutritional (brewer's) yeast and other foods (check the labels), as well as vitamin supplements.

Vitamin D: Vegans should have a reliable source of vitamin D. A supplement may be needed for vegans who get little sunlight.

Calcium: Studies have shown that vegetarians absorb and retain more calcium from foods than non-vegetarians. Vegetable greens such as spinach, kale and broccoli, and some legumes and soybean products are good sources of calcium.

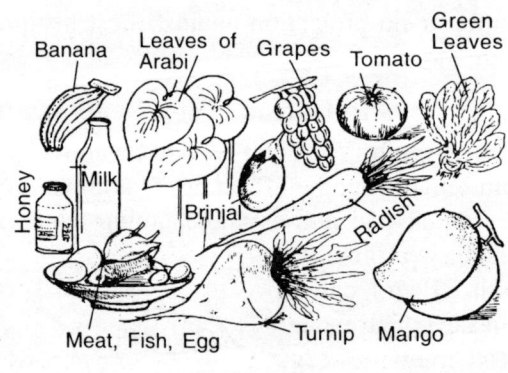

Zinc: It is needed for growth and development. Good plant sources include grains, nuts and legumes. Care should be taken in selecting supplements containing no more than 15-18 mg zinc because supplements containing 50 mg or more may lower HDL ("good") cholesterol in some people.

Tips for Vegetarians

- Vegetarian diets of any type should include a wide variety of foods and enough calories to meet your energy needs.
- Keep your intake of sweets and fatty foods to a minimum. These foods are low in nutrient density.
- Choose whole or unrefined grain products when possible, or use fortified or enriched cereal products.
- Use a variety of fruits and vegetables, including foods that are good sources of vitamins A and C.
- If you use milk or dairy products, choose skim or low-fat or non-fat varieties.
- Eggs are considered all right for most vegetarian diets, but one must use it with moderation. Because eggs have a high cholesterol content (213 mg per yolk), monitor your use of eggs as you try to limit your cholesterol intake to no more than 300 mg per day.

Combining Foods for Balanced Nutrition

Vegans must plan their diet especially well because no single fruit, vegetable or grain contains the nutritionally complete protein food that is found in meat, milk and eggs. Beans, nuts, peas and many other vegetarian foods contain large amounts of protein. However, these foods must be eaten in particular combinations to provide the body with nutritionally complete protein. For example, beans and rice eaten together provide complete protein, but neither food does this when eaten in isolation.

To obtain calcium, vegans must eat sesame seeds or certain green leafy vegetables, such as broccoli or spinach. The iron and other elements in these vegetables are absorbed better when combined with vitamin C so squeezing a lime on the dish makes it easier to absorb the nutrients.

Healthful Soy

For thousands of years, populations throughout much of the world consumed soybeans without realizing that this bean has some miraculous health properties. Chinese and Japanese cuisine is replete with recipes that incorporate this wonder food.

Today, soy has become the centre of a lot of attention. Researchers are studying the compounds found in soy that may not only help reduce the risk of some diseases, such as heart disease, osteoporosis and cancer, but also help alleviate the symptoms of menopause. Doctors found that when animal protein coming from meat was replaced by textured soybean protein in patients suffering with elevated blood cholesterol, there was a significant reduction in blood cholesterol levels. Further research discovered that the protein from soybeans contains a unique amino acid composition, which seems to produce the cholesterol lowering effect.

For vegetarians, this food takes on a special relevance since it compensates for the nutritional loss of a vegetarian diet.

Listed below are some of the more common soy foods in the market today.

Green Vegetable Soybeans

These large soybeans are harvested when the beans are still green and taste sweet. They can be served as a snack or a main vegetable dish, after boiling in slightly salted water for 15 to 20 minutes. They are high in protein and fibre and contain no cholesterol.

Meat Alternatives

Meat alternatives (also called meat analogs) are non-meat foods made from soy protein and other ingredients mixed together to simulate various kinds of meat. Usually, they can be used the same way as the foods they replace.

Soy Cheese

It is made from soy milk. It can substitute for sour cream or cream cheese and can be found in a variety of flavours in natural-food stores.

Soy Flour

Soy flour is made from roasted soybeans that are ground into a fine powder. To turn a normal wheat flour into a protein packed one, mix in soyflour which can easily be made out of soy bean. Soyflour is gluten-free, so yeast-raised breads made with soy flour are more dense in texture. Replace ¼ to 1/3 of the flour called for in a recipe (for muffins, cakes, cookies, pancakes and quick breads) with soy flour.

Soy Granules

Soy granules are similar to soy flour, except that the soybeans have been toasted and cracked into coarse pieces, rather than the fine powder of soy flour. Soy grits can be used as a substitute for flour in some recipes. High in protein, soy grits can be cooked together with other grains.

Soy Protein Isolates

When protein is removed from defatted flakes, the result is soy protein isolates. They contain the most amount of protein of all soy products.

Textured Soy Flour

It is made by running defatted soy flour through an extrusion cooker, which allows for many different forms and sizes. When hydrated, it has a chewy texture. It is widely used as a meat extender. Textured soy flour contains about 70 percent protein and retains most of the bean's dietary fibre. It is sold dried in granular and chunk style.

Soy Sauce

This is a dark brown liquid made from soybeans that have undergone a fermenting process. Soy sauces have a salty taste, but are lower in sodium than traditional table salt. It is extensively used in Chinese cuisine.

Soy Yoghurt

It is made from soymilk. Its creamy texture makes it an easy substitute for sour cream or cream cheese. Soy yoghurt can be found in a variety of flavours in natural-food stores.

Soybeans, Whole

As soybeans mature in the pod, they ripen into a hard, dry bean. Most soybeans are yellow, but there are brown and black varieties. Whole soybeans (an excellent source of protein and dietary fibre) can be cooked and used in sauces, stews and soups. Whole soybeans that have been soaked can be roasted for snacks.

Soy Milk, Soy Beverages

Soybeans, soaked, ground fine and strained, produce a fluid called soybean milk, which is a good substitute for cow's milk. Plain, unfortified soy milk is an excellent source of high-quality protein and B-vitamins.

Soy Nuts

Roasted soy nuts are whole soybeans that have been soaked in water and then baked until browned. Soy nuts can be found in a variety of flavours, including chocolate. High in protein and isoflavones, soy nuts are similar in texture and flavour to peanuts.

Soy Oil and Products

Soy oil is the natural oil extracted from whole soybeans. Soy oil is cholesterol-free and high in polyunsaturated fat. It also is used to make margarine and shortening.

Tofu and Tofu Products

Tofu, also known as soybean curd, is a soft cheese-like food made by curdling fresh, hot soymilk with a coagulant. Tofu is a bland product that easily absorbs the flavours of other ingredients with which it is cooked. Tofu is rich in high-quality protein and B-vitamins and low in sodium.

Firm tofu (easy to stir fry or grill) is dense and solid and can be cubed and served in soups. Firm tofu is higher in protein, fat and calcium than other forms of tofu. Soft tofu is good for recipes that call for blended tofu. Silken tofu is a creamy product and can be used as a replacement for sour cream in many dip recipes.

A good diet can also be an interesting and tasty one, provided one can be creative about putting it together. All one needs to remember is that we should not become slaves to our taste buds, which may learn to appreciate the rich and spicy stuff more than the nutritious one. Imaginative experimentation with various food combinations and learning the art of calorie balancing could work wonders with one's fitness and health.

■ ■

2. Foods That Heal

Much before scientists created pharmacological chemicals and produced medicines to heal human beings our forefathers used herbs and food for curing all kinds of ailments. Most of these herbs are returning with a vigour in modern times. For thousands of years, food has been regarded as potent medicine. But in the last century, pharmaceutical drugs have taken over as magic cures, making us forget much of our rich heritage in the medicinal uses of food. One of the reasons that caused the tilt towards pharmaceutical drugs is the quick effect in curing an ailment. It is only in the recent years to avoid side effects of drugs that attention was diverted to alternative medicines and food cures.

The medical profession's romance with food is ancient. There are numerous prescriptions on stone and papyrus dating back to 4000 B.C. that list foods as cures for most common diseases. The father of modern medicine, Hippocrates, proclaimed food and medicine inseparable. The great Jewish physician-philosopher Maimonides of the 12th century in his treatise on asthma included recipes for chicken soup as remedies. For 40 centuries Oriental culture has regarded food and medicine as indistinguishable.

A lot of research is currently going on, around the globe, regarding the veracity of the ancient beliefs and scientists worldwide are routinely discovering remarkable medicines in our food. That such food chemicals can alleviate and prevent disease was confirmed by leading scientists and physicians who have been involved in the research for the past two decades. They have found that medicines that bring relief to people in most ailments can be found in everyday foods.

With the new scientific information, you can control your own health. By making changes in your diet, you may prevent and alleviate both acute and chronic maladies. Many common ailments such as infections, heart disease, high blood pressure, cancer, constipation and other gastrointestinal diseases, ulcers, arthritis, skin disorders, headaches, low energy, and insomnia can be cured by eating the right kind of food.

Food has an unimaginable range of elements which covers natural laxatives, tranquillisers, beta blockers, antibiotics, anticoagulants, antidepressants, painkillers, cholesterol reducers, anti-inflammatory agents, hypotensives, analgesics, decongestants, digestive expectorants, anti-motion sickness agents, cancer inhibitors, antioxidants, contraceptives, vasodilators and vaso-contrictors, anti-cavity agents, anti-ulcerative agents, insulin regulators, to name a few.

Research shows that foods and their individual constituents perform in similar manner as modern drugs, and sometimes better, without the dreaded side effects. For example, sugar works even when antibiotics fail to heal a wound. Yoghurt, a common fare in our diets, is better at boosting immunity than a drug designed for that purpose and cures diarrhoea more quickly than a standard anti-diarrhoeal drug. Surprisingly, it contains agents that are a stronger antibiotic than penicillin. Onion raises beneficial HDL cholesterol levels in the blood more effectively than most prescription heart medicine including the latest wonder drugs. The compounds contained in garlic can match aspirin in preventing blood clots that may lead to heart attacks and strokes.

Fish (notably mackerel) is remarkable in depressing mild high blood pressure. Ginger surpasses medicine in suppressing motion sickness. A couple of tablespoons of sugar at bedtime can put you to sleep, better than some sleeping pills. Red wine knocks off bacteria as effectively as penicillin. These food items have been used by generations before us but we have never paid heed to the natural capacity of food to cure ailments. The new found interest in the healing powers of food have stunned the scientific community. It is also leading to the extraction and synthesis of natural active agents in foods that can be used in concentrated form for therapeutic purposes.

Nutraceuticals

In recent years one has increasingly been exposed to certain new words in connection with food and pharmacy. One of these words is nutraceuticals and the other is phytochemicals.

Nutraceuticals are functional foods that have potentially disease-preventing and health-promoting properties. They are also naturally occurring dietary substances in pharmaceutical dosage forms, thus including "dietary supplements" as well as comparable substances unintended for oral ingestion.

Phytochemicals

These are chemical substances that plants naturally produce to protect themselves against viruses, bacteria and fungi. Tens of thousands of phytochemicals exist in the foods we eat - nearly all of them in fruits and vegetables. They're what give the plants their colour and flavour, they also serve as the plant's defence system against disease and pollutants. They defend us against a lot of diseases. Some examples include allicin in garlic and isoflavones in soy foods.

These nutraceuticals, as they're sometimes called, may help protect against some cancers, heart disease and chronic health conditions. The common cabbage contains phytochemicals called indoles, which are great cancer fighters; onions contain no less than 50 different phytochemicals; and the best of the lot is called allelic sulphide. The capsicum contains capsaicin, a neutraliser of known carcinogens. Citrus fruits and lemons contain monoterpene, a cancer-fighter. Strawberries are full of ellagic aid, another anticarcinogen and the lycopene contained in tomatoes is one of the best phytochemicals, which acts as an antioxidant.

Garlic is Great

Garlic has proved itself as a wonder drug, which can effectively combat bacteria without causing the common side effects noticed in the case of anti-bacterial pharmaceutical medicines. Garlic was once used extensively to treat tuberculosis, a fungal infection. In fact, in the days before manmade antibiotics, garlic was the drug of choice against TB.

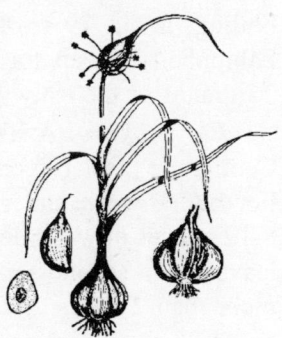

41

The ancient Egyptians worshipped it. Pliny the Elder, a Roman administrator and naturalist living in the 1st century A.D. recommended garlic for no fewer than 61 ailments. Even Louis Pasteur in 1858 put a dollop of garlic in a petri dish and recorded that the bacteria died.

It has been used since time immemorial to cure flatulence. It is also prescribed to lower blood pressure. It forms the base of many medicines for lung disorders and respiratory diseases. Regular intake can also cure skin blemishes and ailments. A paste made of it gives relief from pain caused by the sting of a scorpion.

Garlic contains high amounts of antioxidants, vitamin A, vitamin C, carotene, and selenium and boosts the levels of antioxidant enzymes in the bloodstream. Consuming a couple of cloves of garlic may keep your friends away but they definitely help to protect the neurons from damage.

Green Tea Magic

In China, green tea has been considered a crude medicine for 4,000 years. Researchers have found that green tea protects blood vessels, suppresses cancer, and prolongs life. In recent years, green tea has emerged as a magic combatant against free-radical damage since it contains a variety of antioxidants, including catechin, and is known to lower cholesterol levels and reduce blood clotting.

Brewing Green Tea

There are several methods of brewing green tea for maximum efficacy.

For sencha: After you have brought the kettle to boil allow the water to cool for about 3 minutes. The water should be hot, but not boiling, about 79 to 87 degrees Centigrade (175-190 degrees Fahrenheit). Steep for 1-2 minutes. Do not steep longer than 2 minutes or the tea will become overly astringent.

For gyokuro: A slightly lower temperature 70 to 80 degrees Centigrade (160-175 degrees Fahrenheit). Steep for 2-3 minutes. For both *sencha* and *gyokuro*: use 1 teaspoon of tea for every 8-12 ounces of water depending on your taste. If you use the same leaves for a second serving do it right away. If the leaves sit for more than 2 hours discard them and brew a fresh pot.

Genmai cha: Use the same ratio of tea to water as *sencha* and *gyokuro.* Steep for 1 minute. Water temperature is the same as *sencha* - about 79 to 87 degrees Centigrade (175-190 degrees Fahrenheit).

For matcha: Use 1 level teaspoon of tea to ½ cup of water for medium tea or 2 level teaspoons to ½ cup of water for strong tea. Put *matcha* into a bowl and pour hot (but not boiling) water over the tea. Use a bamboo whisk to whip the tea into a frothy brew. This tea is very potent. For this reason it is not recommended making more than ½ cup (100 ml) for one person per serving.

Gingko and Ginseng

In traditional Oriental medicine ginseng root became known as a 'whole-body tonic'. Of all the herbs of China, ginseng root, since antiquity, has been the most highly prized 'elixir vitae'. Certain herbs like ginkgo, ginseng and amino acids like L-carnitine prevent the degenerative condition of the brain and other vital organs. These elements are also known to have healing powers for the brain. They help in many ways like improving decision-making abilities, increasing attention span and mnemonic capacity. It is for this reason that many of the memory improving drugs available in the market, contain ginseng or ginkgo.

One of the herbs known for its influence on the brain, especially the memory, is ginkgo biloba. Ginkgo increases the rate at which information is transmitted at the nerve-cell level. Ginkgo increases circulation, especially the circulation in tiny blood vessels, such as those in the brain. It dilates blood vessels by releasing a vessel-relaxing factor. This characteristic improves oxygen and nutrient delivery to the brain, and is one of the reasons that ginkgo has a reputation for increasing memory.

The leaves of the Ginkgo biloba tree, also known as the maidenhair tree, have been used for more than 5,000 years for medicinal purposes. It's one of the most widely used herbal extracts in Europe, and has been approved by the German government to treat symptoms of ageing, including cognitive disorders.

Ginkgo has been shown to have the following effects:
- Improve overall cognitive function and sharpen mental focus.

- Prevent and treat symptoms of dementia.
- Slow the progression of Alzheimer's in its early stages, and progressive decrease in symptoms of Alzheimer's disease.
- Treat "cerebral insufficiency", a slow decline in mental function associated with ageing and characterized by such symptoms as impaired concentration and memory, confusion, and mood disorders.

As a potent antioxidant, ginkgo helps protect against cellular damage.

Potent Oyster

Amongst all the foods that have been hailed as aphrodisiacs, oysters hold pride of place as a key to potency and fertility. Unlike most aphrodisiacs, oysters have the doctors' backing because they are nature's most concentrated packages of zinc. They are richer in zinc than any other food by far. 3 ounces of raw oysters have 63 mgms of zinc. Experts say it's tough to get enough zinc unless you eat oysters. What happens to males who don't eat enough zinc? They don't mature sexually; their gonads shrink up. Also, normal males with zinc deficiencies fail to produce enough male hormone testosterone and sperm, and can become infertile or impotent.

Citrus Cure

In 1985, Canadian researchers reported that vitamin C doses (1000 milligrams a day) helped prevent stomach cancer, but little more than 3 fluid ounces of orange juice daily (containing 37 mg of vitamin C) was twice as likely to depress the chances of developing stomach cancer.

Probably the most well-known antioxidant, vitamin C helps minimize free radical damage to the neurological system. In the presence of hesperidin, a bioflavonoid, vitamin C is an even more powerful antioxidant. It also protects other antioxidants in the body, such as vitamin E. In addition, vitamin C detoxifies the body, reduces high blood pressure, lowers cholesterol, and fights cancer. Some of the citrus fruits that contain a lot of vitamin C are oranges and gooseberries.

Oranges and Lemons

Oranges are known for their protective effects against various diseases. Rich in vitamins B, C and calcium, they provide quick energy to the body. Oranges are useful in maintaining the digestive organs, kidneys, blood vessels and nervous system. They also prevent gingivitis and pyorrhoea and strengthen the teeth.

The high content of minerals like lime and magnesium, bone building elements, make it very valuable for growth of children. The potash contained in its juice is alkaline in reaction. Because of its quick absorption and utilisation, orange juice is preferred as nutrition during convalescing. The fibre in this fruit acts as a digestive tract cleanser.

Loaded with citric acid and alkaline minerals, they improve the liver functions by increasing the flow of bile. A very effective cure for rheumatism, gout and arthritis, lemons help in dissolving the uric acid. It finds use in curing catarrh, sore throat, cough and diphtheria, also.

Tomato Truths

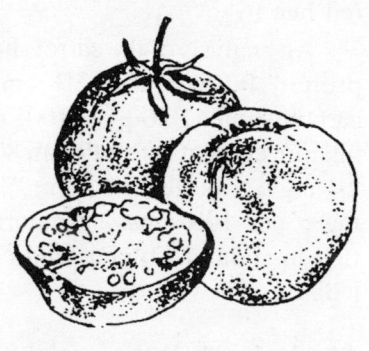

Amongst the various foods that contain antioxidants, tomatoes are known to be full of an element called lycopene. It is actually the substance that gives tomatoes their red colour and, like beta-carotene, lycopene is a member of the carotenoid family.

Research on dietary lycopene suggests that it may lower the risk of heart attack. A five-year study of 48,000 men found that those eating ten servings per week of cooked tomato products had the lowest risk of prostate cancer. Believe it or not, their risk was only one-third that of men eating less than two servings per week. Other studies suggest that lycopene may play a major role in reducing the risk of other cancers, including cancers of the breast, rectum and colon.

While fresh tomatoes are loaded with lycopene, cooking them makes it even easier for your body to use their lycopene. Apparently, as the tomatoes break down when they are cooked, the lycopene is more easily absorbed. Including a little fat will help, too, especially mono saturated fat like olive oil.

Carrot Value

Carrots are probably the most concentrated source of beta-carotene, which, in addition to its possible role as a cancer fighter, may play a key role in preventing the formation of cataracts later in life. Beta-carotene, a source of vitamin a, also may boost your immune system's ability to fight bacterial and viral infections.

Nutritionally the carrot is an extremely rich source of vitamin A. Carotene is converted into vitamin A by the liver and it is stored in the organ. The word carotene has been derived from the word carrot.

Carotenoids-the magic factor contained in all orange coloured vegetables-is the secret of this cure. This benefit is not confined to carrots, it is the primary pigment of all deep-orange and deep-green vegetables. (Green chlorophyll covers up the orange or red hue.)

An analysis of the carrot shows it to consist of moisture 86.0%, protein 0.9%, fat 0.2%, minerals 1.1%, fibre 1.2%, and carbohydrates 10.6% per 100 gms of edible portion. Its mineral and vitamin contents are calcium 80 mg%, phosphorus 530 mg%, iron 2.2 mg%, riboflavin 0.02mg %, niacin 0.6 mg% and vitamin C 3 mg% per 100 gms. Its calorific value is 48. Carrots are also rich in sodium, sulphur and chlorine and they contain traces of iodine.

Medicinal Properties

Carrot is rich in alkaline elements, which purify and revitalise the blood. It nourishes the entire system and helps in the maintenance of the acid alkaline balance in the body. Carrot juice makes a fine health drink for children and adults alike. It strengthens the eyes and keeps the mucous membranes in a healthy condition. It is also beneficial in the treatment of dry and rough skin.

It is absolutely marvellous as a cleanser and prevents tooth decay. Chewing carrots increases saliva production and quickens digestion by supplying the necessary enzymes, minerals and vitamins. Regular intake of carrots prevents the formation of gastric ulcers and other digestive disorders. Its juice is an effective food remedy for ailments like intestinal colic, colitis, appendicitis, peptic ulcers and dyspepsia. An effective cure for constipation, it is one of the few vegetables, that naturally replenish sodium, potassium, magnesium and other minerals during dehydration caused by diarrhoea.

The best sources for anti-cancer carotenoids are apricot (especially the dried kind), broccoli, brussels sprouts, green cabbage, carrots, kale, lettuce, spinach, squash, sweet potatoes and tomatoes.

Cancer-Fighting Crucifers

Cruciferous vegetables like cabbage, broccoli and cauliflower have recently come under a lot of attention mainly for their anti-cancer effects. Broccoli, for instance, is a wonder food, one of the best nutrition bets around. Not only is broccoli high in fibre and vitamin C, it provides folic acid, calcium magnesium and iron. Certain chemicals found in broccoli and related vegetables appear to help prevent lung cancer—even in smokers.

Researchers from the National Institute of Environmental and Health Sciences and their colleagues in China studied people in Shanghai. The people in these Chinese communities eat a lot of cruciferous vegetables. They also smoke a lot, which puts them at higher risk for lung cancer. When the researchers tested the blood levels of the people who smoked and also ate a lot of cruciferous vegetables, they found that these people had a 36 percent lower cancer rate than the smokers who didn't eat the cruciferous vegetables.

Scientists found that if you ate cabbage more than once a week you were only one third as likely to develop colon cancer as someone who never ate cabbage. In other words, one serving of cabbage a week could cut your chances of colon cancer by 66 percent. Even if you ate cabbage once every two or three weeks, the risk dropped by forty percent.

The most effective members of the cruciferous family are: – broccoli, brussels sprouts, cabbage, cauliflower, cress, horseradish, kale, mustard, radish and turnip.

Juice Power

Fruit & Vegetable Juice Therapy

"Let living (natural) food be thy medicine." – Hippocrates made this statement some 2,400 years ago.

These prophetic words are the basis of modern research in the healing power of food. In these simple words, he tried to explain that in raw fruits and vegetables lay the essential drug to control and fight human ailments most effectively.

If the human body is kept free from any toxins or waste products, then it can remain free of disease. Raw fruit juice therapy has proved quite effective in removing toxins from our bodies.

Fruit and vegetable juices may be divided into six main types:

1. From sweet fruits such as prunes and grapes.
2. From sub-acid fruits like apple, plum, pear, peach, apricot and cherry.
3. From acid fruits like orange, lemon, grapefruit, strawberry and pineapple.
4. From vegetable fruits, namely, tomato and cucumber.
5. From green leafy vegetables like cabbage, celery, lettuce, spinach, parsley and watercress.
6. From root vegetables like beetroot, carrot, onion, potato and radish.

It is believed that fruit juices stir up toxins and acids in the body, thereby stimulating the eliminative processes. Vegetable juices, on the other hand, carry away toxic matter in a gentler way. Owing to their differing actions fruit and vegetable juices should not be used at the same time. And not more than three juices should be used in any one mixture.

The following broad rules apply when using mixtures:

- Juices from sweet fruits may be combined with juices of sub-acid fruits, but not with those of acid fruits, vegetable fruits or vegetables.
- Juices from sub-acid fruits may be combined with juices of sweet fruits, or acid fruits, but not with other juices.

- Juices from acid fruits may be combined with those of sub-acid fruits or vegetable fruits, but not with other juices.
- Juices from vegetable fruits may be combined with those of acid fruits or of green leafy vegetables, but not with other juices.
- Juices from green leafy vegetables may be combined with those of vegetable fruits or of the root vegetable, but not with other juices.
- Juices from root vegetables may be combined with those of green leafy vegetables, but not with other juices.

A proper selection of juices in treating a particular ailment is very essential. Thus, for instance, juices of carrot, cucumber, cabbage and other vegetables are very valuable in asthma, arthritis and skin disease, but orange juice can aggravate their symptoms by increasing the amount of mucus.

The Beneficial Effects of a Few Common Fruits & Vegetables

Apple: A rich source of sorbitol, a type of sugar used to create energy for the body and as a mild laxative. Apples also contain polyphenols, antioxidants thought to counteract viruses.

Beet: Loaded with vitamins C and E, beta-carotene and magnesium. Beet juice is high in potassium and folic acid. Beetroot juice is a potent liver cleanser. It helps to purify the blood and remove toxins. Raw beetroot juice helps promote normal bowel movements and prevents constipation. It also helps strengthen blood vessels, improve blood circulation and reduce cholesterol.

Blueberry and Cranberry: Juices from both these fruits are thought to aid in treating urinary tract infections.

Cantaloupe: Thought to possess anti-coagulative properties, which thin the blood and are believed to aid in the prevention of heart attacks and strokes.

Carrot: Known to be rich in beta-carotene and potassium, as well as the antioxidants glutathione and phthalide (both considered anti-cancerous).

Celery: Rich in sodium and potassium, celery also contains several anti-cancerous antioxidants.

Cherry: Traditionally thought to relieve pain associated with gout.

Lemon: Traditionally lemon has been used as an appetite stimulant and for instigating digestive juice activity as well as the flow of saliva.

Orange: Rich in vitamin C, potassium and a number of other key vitamins and nutrients.

Papaya: Loaded with potassium and magnesium. It also contains papain, a substance thought to have anti-ulcer effects.

Parsley: Considered to be the most effective treatment of bad breath. Although yet unproven, parsley is also said to aid functions of the kidney and enhance eyesight.

Peach: Rich in potassium and also thought to contain a mild laxative.

Pineapple: Pineapple juice contains the enzyme bromelain, an anti-inflammatory agent which can reduce swelling associated with tooth extractions and sore throats.

Radish: Excellent for thinning down mucous and clearing sinus. It also helps in clearing blocked nose and mucous related migraine etc. Radish juice helps to reduce gas formation and indigestion. It is beneficial in reducing phlegm and curing sore throats caused due to phlegm. Its juice helps in detoxification and cleanses the system.

Spinach: Rich in iron, oxalic acid (which aids constipation but causes kidney stones), vitamin C, potassium and calcium.

Recent Research on Food Power

One of the modern findings that have changed the entire concept about health and food are body hormones called prostaglandins. These hormones trigger a range of the body's biochemical processes e.g. they can cause pain, inflammation, skin disorders, sluggish blood, and infertility, among other things. Other groups of prostaglandins can protect the stomach from noxious chemicals and intestinal damage.

Scientific breakthroughs have shown that food chemicals get into the brain and impact neurotransmitters, thus affecting the state of our mind and mood. Certain foods have a considerable effect on the release of prostaglandins and have been found to boost immunity against a horde of viruses and diseases caused by them.

Onions and the Heart

Onions have been used for 5,000 years to cure virtually everything under the sun. Researchers have found that onion has a boosting effects on HDL (good) cholesterol. It has been found that cooking destroys this capacity of boosting the HDL, which is best derived from raw onions. Also,

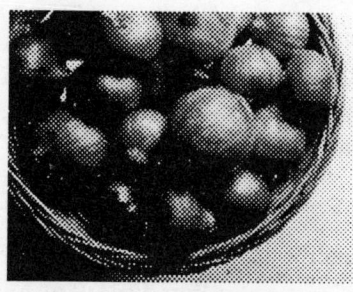

the active agent is one that gives onion its strong taste. The major effect comes from the hotter white and yellow onions; mild red onions don't possess the same effect. The stronger the onion taste, the sharper the elevation of HDLs.

Onion possesses a vigorous concoction of chemicals that perform complex chemotherapy on the cardio-vascular system. Onions contain a compound known to lower blood pressure. The onion also contains adenosine and other chemicals that keep platelets from sticking together. Besides, the onion works on another function of the blood; it revs up the body's fibrinolytic, or blood clot-dissolving, system. Just as some onion chemicals keep platelets from getting together, others actively work to dissolve clots as they form. Onions, both cooked and raw, contain chemicals that promote clot break up.

Studies in Massachusetts shows that men with high blood levels of fibrinogen (the basic substance that causes clots) are more likely to suffer strokes and coronary and artery disease. Thus, researcher say, too much fibrinogen in your blood maybe as hazardous as high blood pressure. Onions can effectively combat high fibrinogen.

A string of subsequent studies showed that boiled, raw, and dried as well as fried onions could also partially clear blood of the ill effects of dietary fat. That is why it makes good sense to top your hamburger with a slab of raw onion or stir up a few onions with your meat preparations.

Barley and Oats

In a study conducted by scientists who tracked 11,000 vegetarians and non-vegetarians for 7 years, it was found that death rates were much lower among the vegetarians.

Do specific factors in vegetables build a body less vulnerable to disease? Tests have shown some distinctive differences. Vegetarians have markedly lower blood cholesterol, especially the detrimental LDL type, and we all know that lower cholesterol cuts the risk of heart attacks.

Dramatic new evidence confirms that reducing destructive LDL type and raising HDL (good type) cholesterol can also help unclog damaged coronary arteries.

In a startling discovery, experts who conducted studies on the fibre intake of vegetarians noticed that when diabetics ate high fibre foods, not only did their blood sugar and insulin improve, their blood cholesterol and blood pressure also fell remarkably. But their triglycerides – another type of fat – went up. This made them conclude that the added fibre could be the main factor that was pushing down blood cholesterol.

This brought about the hypothesis that fibre deficiency is the prime cause of modern ills and that fibre can cure or prevent almost anything that ails you, including diabetes, coronary artery disease, high blood pressure, obesity, haemorrhoids, varicose veins, diverticular disease, hiatus hernia, gall stones, constipation, irritable bowel syndrome, appendicitis and cancer, especially of the colon.

The knowledge that fibres are good for health dates back to the classical Greeks. In the 19th century America, a vegetarian preacher, Sylvester Graham said the primary reason vegetables, fruits, legumes, and grains are healthful is the high content of fibre in them.

And what could be a better source for fibre than barley and oats? In rural India most people consume roti made of bajra, jowar and makai, and have a much healthier and disease-free constitution that the urban lot who eat roti made of refined wheat flour or, worse, white bread.

The Yin Yang Therapy of Chillies

If you have a cold, build a fire in your stomach. This funny remedy has its roots in the ancient medical concept of balancing opposites. In ancient Greco-Roman medicine, every physician worth his salt knew that if you had phlegm, characterizing a "cold disorder", the treatment of choice was "something hot". The traditional Yin Yang theory of therapeutics calls for hot pungent "Yang" spices to treat "cold Yin" respiratory diseases.

Hippocrates prescribed vinegar and pepper as respiratory drugs. The great Roman physician Galen favoured the use of garlic for chest pain. In the middle ages, mustard was a potion used against asthma, coughs and chest congestion. The well-known 12th century Jewish physician, Maimonides, who was an expert on asthma, recommended spicy chicken soup for that condition and "the stirring up and ejection of pulmonary phlegm".

In 1802 the distinguished English physician Herberden recommended garlic and mustard seeds, amongst other agents, to treat asthma. Oriental medicine uses capsicum peppers, black pepper, mustard, garlic, turmeric and other spices to treat cold, sinusitis, bronchitis and asthma. Russians use horseradish to treat colds. Hot foods have been used to treat pulmonary diseases since antiquity. It was found that ancient Egyptian medical writings recommended mustard in respiratory therapy.

In parts of the world where the cuisine is hot, pulmonary disease rates are low. Britain has a high rate of respiratory problems because of the cold and damp weather coupled with the bland dietary habits followed by most Brits.

All this led to a brilliant scientific research by a modern medical theorist and pharmaceutical expert, leading him to some fascinating investigations of chilli peppers.

To know how chillies can actually remove phlegm, you have to know a little about the movement of this blocker of respiratory system. Normally the journey of mucous in the lungs is so subtle that you are not conscious of the routine clearance that pushes mucous up out of the lungs and to the back of the throat, where you swallow it. Rhythmically propelling the mucous along through breathing passages are cilia, tiny hair like projections on cells. All goes well if the mucous is thin enough for the cilia to move. But if the mucous thickens, it is difficult for the cilia to move it. Experts discovered that chillies, just like modern drugs, have a common action: they invariably affect the viscosity and consequent movement of mucous in the lungs.

Thus, critical to lung function is the proper consistency, and regular removal of secretions. The ancients discovered that certain pungent foods possessed so called mucokinetic (moving mucous) agents that thin, regulate, or propel the mucous out of the lungs. Modern drugs that promote the removal of sputum from the respiratory system are described as mucokinetic. It is this mucokinetic effect that explains the pharmacological secrets of hot pungent spices. They literally thin down the lung's secretions so they can be coughed up or normally expelled. It appears that hot spicy foods may also act as a preventive therapy for bronchitis.

One of the most effective chest medications is garlic. Garlic may be an even more potent anti-congestant when combined with vitamin C because vitamin C may help break down Alliin, a major flavouring agent in garlic. Crushing or cutting garlic cloves cause a rapid conversion to allicin.

Fish Formula

For a long time now, research has been done on fat and its effects on the heart. We know that too much fat will clog and stiffen our arteries, bringing forth drastic effects that choke off blood to the brain and harm the heart. Whether your arteries are wrecked and your body suffers considerable other problems may depend on the chemical make up of the fat and its consequent disposition by the body. But animal fats are very different from the ones in fish.

Scientists were perplexed by the fact that Eskimos had virtually no heart disease and yet ate a high fat diet of blubber and seal meat; their blood cholesterol levels, especially among Alaskan Eskimos, were fairly high, only slightly lower than that of Americans, Danes, and others who were dropping dead from heart attacks. Research showed that Eskimo blood is not as sticky and does not clot as readily.

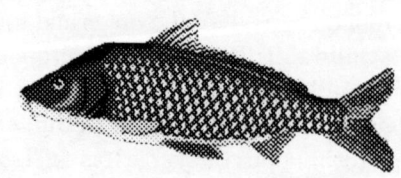

The same phenomenon shows up among families in Japanese fishing villages who are also remarkably free of heart disease. They found that the strange phenomenon was rooted in the fact that the Eskimos loaded themselves with a unique oil found in seafood. They typically devour 13 ounces of seafood every day, all of it heavily packed with molecular chains of fatty acids called omega-3's. In contrast, the fat or oil in land plants and meat from animals raised on such plants are dominated by omega-6 fatty acids that are broken down differently in the body.

An excess of omega-6 provokes the cells to frantic activity, causing the production of excesses of hyperactive prostaglandins and similar hormones that wreak havoc on the body.

Fish oils may protect against thrombosis – clots that block off blood. Cancer, asthma, rheumatoid arthritis, lupus, psoriasis, allergies, immune inflammatory disorders, headaches, high blood pressure and multiple sclerosis are all disorders related to over enthusiastic production of prostaglandins. Fish oils, by curbing prostaglandin formation, may control the underlying metabolic mechanisms that set off these diseases too.

Nutrition experts at UT Southwestern Medical Center in Dallas say older adults who eat just one serving of fatty fish a week can lower their risk of a fatal heart attack by up to 44 percent, compared to people who don't eat fish at all.

But if you prefer your fish fried, you're not getting the benefit. The high heat from frying changes the structure of the beneficial fatty acids so they no longer have the same effect on the body besides the negative effect of all that oil, used for frying, on your body. Fatty fish like salmon, tuna, sardines, mackerel and herring are most beneficial because they have the highest levels of the omega-3 fatty acids that prevent heart disease. These fatty acids are important for growth and development, but they're not manufactured within the human body. Leaner fish like cod and flounder don't have as much omega-3 and are less beneficial. Nutrition experts suggest you bake or grill fish to preserve the health benefits and recommend eating at least two servings of fish every week to help prevent heart disease.

Yoghurt Benefits

Yoghurt or curd, as it is popularly called, has been a normal part of Indian diet. The derivatives of curd such as buttermilk and lassi have been immensely popular, both in the Southern and the Northern parts of the country. A lot of Indian recipes also require the addition of curd, especially in meat preparations. Grandmothers recommended the intake of curd and rice whenever a person suffered from diarrhoea. The lactic microbes, which 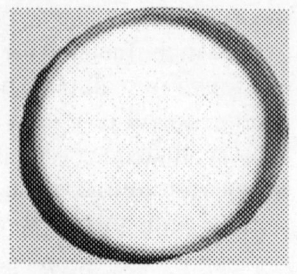 are contained in the curd, are known to retard the bad consequences of intestinal putrefaction.

There's evidence that yoghurt battles bacteria in humans. The longevity factor connected with yoghurt has also been a matter of research. In 1986 French scientists at the National Institute of Health and Medical Research in Paris discovered the possibility that yoghurt might somehow help ward off human breast cancer. They compared the diets of two groups of women: 1,010 women with breast cancer and a comparable group of women without breast cancer. There was an outstanding difference in the diet of women belonging to the two groups, those women who ate yoghurt the most had the lowest risk of breast cancer, and the risk decreased as yoghurt consumption increased.

In another breakthrough, scientists found that the people of Finland had a very low rate of colon cancer although they consumed a diet high in meat, fat, protein and low in fibre. Studies showed that the Finns also consumed a lot of dairy products, mainly yoghurt. It was deduced that the yoghurt could have a hand in keeping the colon cancer rates extraordinarily low.

Yoghurt is created by the active action of a variety of bacteria, usually from a large family called lactobacillus. When mixed in milk, these bacterial strains proliferate, causing the milk to curdle or ferment (taking on a sour taste) and thicken or coagulate. These bacteria create unique metabolic compounds that alter the chemistry of the milk, and bring about a beneficial impact on human physiology and disease. The strain of bacteria used determines the character of the yoghurt or fermented milk and its peculiar health benefit.

Nowhere is food's healing power better illustrated than by vegetarians. They have lower rates of cancer, heart disease, stroke, and a number of other chronic diseases than meat eaters.

At first one explanation was that they eat less saturated fat. That evolved into the theory that maybe the higher fibre foods they eat counteract some of the effects of the fat. Then it began to dawn that maybe vegetables, fruits, legumes, nuts, and other plant foods containing pharmacologically protective agents – the minor dietary constituents – are potent enough in counteracting cellular assaults that foster disease.

The Healing Power

Apple

- A good heart medicine
- Lowers blood cholesterol
- Lowers blood pressure
- Stabilises blood sugar
- Dampens appetite
- Packed with chemicals that block cancer in animals
- Apple juice kills infectious viruses

Banana & Plantain

- Prevents and heals ulcers
- Lowers blood cholesterol

Barley

- Lowers blood cholesterol
- May inhibit cancer
- Improves bowel function
- Relieves constipation

Beans

Includes black beans, black-eyed peas, chickpeas, faba beans, kidney beans, lentils, lima beans, split peas, pinto beans, white Great Northern, navy and white beans, and common baked beans.

- Reduces bad type blood cholesterol
- Contains chemicals that inhibit cancer
- Controls insulin and blood sugar
- Lowers blood pressure
- Regulates functions of the colon

- Prevents and cures constipation
- Prevents haemorrhoids and other bowel problems

Cabbage
- Lowers the risk of cancer, especially of the colon
- Prevents and heals ulcers (juice especially)
- Stimulates the immune system
- Kills bacteria and viruses
- Fosters growth

Carrot
- Believed useful in blocking cancer, especially smoking related cancer, including lung
- Lowers blood cholesterol
- Prevents constipation

Cauliflower
- Reduces risk of cancer, especially colon and stomach

Coffee
- Improves mental performance
- Relieves asthma (broncho-dilator)
- Relieves hay fever
- Boosts physical energy
- Prevents cavities
- Contains chemicals that block cancer in animals
- Elevates your mood

Corn
- Contains chemicals that prevent cancer
- Lowers risk of certain cancers, heart disease and cavities
- Oil lowers blood cholesterol

Brinjal
- Protects arteries from cholesterol damage
- Contains chemicals that prevent cancer in animals
- Contains chemicals that prevent convulsions

Fig

- Fights cancer
- Juice kills bacteria
- Juice kills roundworms
- Aids digestion

Fish

- Thins the blood
- Protects arteries from damage
- Inhibits blood clots (anti-thrombotic)
- Reduces blood triglycerides
- Lowers bad-type blood cholesterol
- Lowers blood pressure
- Reduces risk of heart attack and stroke
- Lessens symptoms of rheumatoid arthritis
- Reduces the risk of lupus
- Ameliorates migraine headaches
- Acts as an anti-inflammatory agent
- Regulates immune system
- Prevents cancer in animals
- Relieves bronchial asthma
- Combats early kidney disease
- Increases mental energy

Garlic

- Fights infections
- Contains cancer-preventive chemicals
- Thins the blood (anti-coagulant)
- Reduces blood pressure, cholesterol, triglycerides
- Stimulates the immune system
- Prevents and relieves chronic bronchitis
- Acts as an expectorant and decongestant

Ginger

- Prevents motion sickness
- Thins the blood

- Lowers the blood cholesterol
- Prevents cancer in animals

Grape
- Inactivates viruses
- Thwarts tooth decay
- Rich in compounds that block cancer in animals

Green chillies
- Excellent medicine for the lungs
- Acts as an expectorant
- Prevents and alleviates chronic bronchitis and emphysema
- Acts as a decongestant
- Helps dissolve blood clots
- Kills pain
- Induces euphoria

Honey
- Kills bacteria
- Disinfects wounds and sores
- Reduces perception of pain
- Alleviates asthma
- Soothes sore throats
- Calms the nerves, induces sleep
- Relieves diarrhoea

Lemon and lime
- Prevents and cures scurvy
- Contains chemicals that block cancer

Milk
- Prevents osteoporosis
- Fights infections especially diarrhoea
- Modifies upset stomach from harsh foods and drugs
- Prevents peptic ulcers
- Prevents cavities
- Prevents chronic bronchitis

- Increases mental energy
- Lowers high blood pressure
- Lowers blood cholesterol
- Inhibits certain cancers

Mushroom

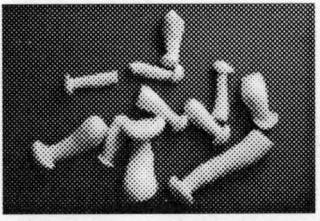

- Thins the blood
- Prevents cancer in animals
- Lowers blood cholesterol
- Stimulates the immune system
- Inactivates viruses

Oats

- An excellent heart medicine
- Lowers blood cholesterol
- Regulates blood sugar
- Contains compounds that prevent cancer in animals
- Combats inflammation of the skin
- Acts as a laxative

Olive Oil

- Reduces bad LDL cholesterol
- Raises good HDL cholesterol
- Thins the blood
- Contains chemicals that retard cancer and ageing
- Lowers risk of death from all causes
- Lowers blood pressure

Onion

- A multi-faceted heart-blood medicine
- Boosts beneficial HDL cholesterol
- Thins the blood
- Lowers total blood cholesterol
- Retards blood clotting
- Regulates blood sugar
- Kills bacteria

- Relieves bronchial congestion
- Blocks cancer in animals

Orange

- Combats certain viruses
- Lowers blood cholesterol
- Fights arterial plaque
- Lowers the risk of certain cancers

Pea

- High in contraceptive agents
- Rich in compounds that prevent cancer in animals
- Prevents appendicitis
- Lowers blood cholesterol

Rice

- Lowers blood pressure
- Fights diarrhoea
- Prevents kidney stones
- Clears up psoriasis (A skin disease)
- Contains chemicals that prevent cancer

Seaweed or Kelp

- Kills bacteria
- Blocks cancer in animals
- Boosts immune system
- Heals ulcers
- Reduces blood cholesterol
- Lowers blood pressure
- Prevents strokes
- Thins the blood

Soybean

- Excellent cardiovascular medicine
- Lowers blood cholesterol
- Prevents and dissolves gallstones
- Reduces triglycerides

- Regulates the bowels
- Relieves constipation
- Regulates blood sugar
- Lowers cancer risk
- Replaces oestrogen
- Promotes contraception

Sugar

- Acts as a tranquilliser
- Relieves anxiety and stress
- Induces relaxation and sleep
- Boosts concentration in some persons
- Acts as an antidepressant
- Kills bacteria
- Heals wounds

Tea

- Reduces cavities
- Destroys bacteria and viruses
- Fights infections
- Contains chemicals that prevent cancer in animals
- Lowers blood pressure
- Strengthens capillaries
- Retards atherosclerosis (hardening of arteries)
- Acts as a mild sedative (decaffeinated)

Wheat Bran

- Relieves constipation
- Prevents diverticular disease, varicose veins, haemorrhoids, and hiatal hernia
- Improves general bowel functioning
- Linked to lower rates of colon cancer

Wine

- Kills bacteria and viruses
- Prevents heart disease (if taken in very moderate doses)
- Raises good HDL blood cholesterol

- Rich in chemicals that prevent cancer in animals

Yoghurt

- Kills bacteria
- Prevents and treats intestinal infections, including diarrhoea
- Lowers blood cholesterol
- Boosts immune system
- Improves bowel functioning
- Contains compounds that prevent ulcers
- Has anti-cancer activity

The following table shows a few common ailments and the food items that can help in curing the problem.

Disease	Healing food	Protective food
Acne	Cucumber, Honey Suckle (Flower), Carrots, Watermelon	Same as Healing Food
Anaemia	Red meats like Beef, Leafy Vegetables	Same as Healing Food
Blocked Nose	Peppermint, Spinach	
Cancer	–	Cruciferous vegetables such as Broccoli, Cauliflower
Cholera	Hyacinth Beans, Pepper	
Constipation	Potato, Banana, Walnut, Almond, Sesame Oil	Same as Healing Food
Cough	Banana, Pine nut, Ginger	–
Fever	Rambutan	–
Food Poisoning / Diarrhoea	Ginger, Spring Onion, Garlic, Apple, Lychee, Chestnut, Cinnamon, Tea, Rice, Hyacinth Beans, Kang Kong, Rambutan	–
Gastric	Milk, Chilli, Sugar Cane Juice	–
Headaches	Celery, Kang Kong, PepperPepper	–

Disease	Healing food	Protective food
High Blood Pressure	Water Chestnut	Same as Healing Food
Indigestion	Orange, Carrot, Hyacinth Beans	–
Kidney Deficiency	Beef, Leafy Vegetables	Same as Healing Food
Kidney Stones	Kiwi Fruit	–
Measles	Chinese Water Chestnut, Ginger	–
Night Blindness/Vision	Carrot, Chrysanthemum (Flowers), Chinese Water Chestnut	Same as Healing Food
Poor Appetite	Cabbage, Potato, Jasmine (Flower), Honey, Rice, Milk, Ginger	–
Rheumatism	Hyacinth Beans, Pepper	–
Shortness of Breath	Lychee	–
Sleeplessness	Kang Kong	Same as Healing Food
Sore Throat	Peppermint, Olive, Ladyfinger	–

Herbs That Cure

The kitchen is a veritable natural pharmacy. Here is a list of herbs and spices that have curative properties:

Basil

In Arabian countries, basil is used as a tea to alleviate menstrual cramps; for that reason, men won't eat anything flavoured with it. In India it is considered the "king of herbs" and it can also be found in Mexico, South America, and the Caribbean. It is an excellent breath freshener, has blood pressure lowering components, and it also has been used successfully, as a tea, to combat the nausea from chemotherapy.

Bay Leaf

In Antigua, bay leaf is used in teas with peppermint and hot chocolate to ward off colds, flu, and bad omens. In Greece, bay leaves were made into crowns to honour poets and soldiers. It may help diabetics as in test tube studies it breaks down blood sugar three times faster than insulin. Boiled bay leaves may be used as a poultice on the chest to relieve cough. Bay leaves are also used in cooking beans to improve their digestibility.

Chives

They're a member of the onion family and contain sulphur. They've been linked to reducing blood pressure and cholesterol, and to prevent cancer. Chives should not be cooked, but snipped or sliced and used raw as a garnish.

Coriander/cilantro *(leaf and seed)*

Both the leaves and seeds are used in cooking. During the Han dynasty in China, the leaves were considered as aphrodisiacs. In India it is supposed to "cool" a hot stomach, banish intestinal gas, and aid digestion. Two tablespoons of chopped coriander leaf should be eaten as soon as indigestion hits, or sprinkled on the food for prevention. In ayurvedic medicine, an after-meal digestive aid is made by combining a teaspoon each of coriander and fennel seeds, toasting them in a dry skillet for about two minutes, until fragrant, and adding a pinch of salt. Chew well. As a remedy for rashes, mash the fresh leaves and apply as and "anti-fire, or anti-pitta" poultice, followed by a cup of coriander seed tea (2 tsp in 1 cup boiling water, 7 minutes).

Dill seed

Dill was used in early Greece and Rome as an air freshener; the seeds were burned as incense. In the early US colonies it was called "meeting seed" because it was chewed for breath freshener during long church meetings. Tea made from dill seed helps soothe upset stomach. Dill seed is also rich in calcium, with 100 mg in a tablespoon. For chapped skin on hands and spit nails, make dill seed oil: warm ½ cup olive, grape seed, or canola oil, then pour into a bottle with 2 tablespoons of dill seed. Steep, covered, for one week; then strain, and use on hands and feet right after washing.

Fennel seed

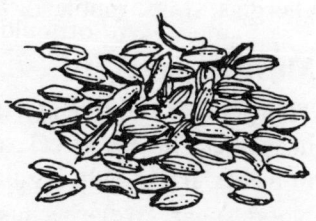

This is a classic Greek and Middle Eastern remedy for intestinal gas. They can be used as a tea, or chewed directly after a meal, as they often are in India. The tea is often used to combat infant colic. Hot fennel tea helps respiratory congestion, and three cups a day help nursing mothers produce more milk.

Garlic

This is the king of all medicinal herbs. Its use goes back at least 5,000 years. In China, it was prescribed raw for colds; Chinese prisoners were required to eat raw garlic every morning to maintain their health. Egyptian slaves were fed garlic and onions to make them strong enough to build the pyramids. It was thought to ward off vampires and evil spirits. Science has vindicated folklore. An average clove of garlic contains substances equivalent to 100,000 units of penicillin (about 1/5 the average dose), without its side effects. It can prevent various types of cancer (stomach, skin, breast, oesophageal, and colon) and prevent cancer cells from reproducing. It reduces cholesterol and high blood pressure, but you need to eat one to three fresh cloves per day for at least three months before positive results are seen. It may even help regulate blood sugar for diabetics. Most of the benefits are from the raw bulb. An Asian remedy consists of a whole bulb of garlic, peeled and minced, and marinated overnight in enough honey to cover. A teaspoon of this honey three times a day has been credited with eliminating colds.

Ginger

Another powerful herb, popular in China, India and Japan for thousands of years, it travelled to the Middle East and Spain, then the West Indies. Ginger ale was first made in Jamaica to help digestive distress. It's an excellent remedy for indigestion and nausea, including motion sickness, and morning sickness. It prevents stomach flu and the nausea associated with chemotherapy. Ginger tea is helpful for headaches, chest congestion, and indigestion. A ginger bath is used in Asia to combat stuffed noses due to allergies, sinus trouble, or colds.

Mustard seed

This popular condiment has been used since prehistory, as well as in ancient Chinese, Greek, and Roman kitchens to prevent rancidity in meats. It can help regulate irregular heartbeat, cholesterol and blood sugar levels because of its magnesium content. Ground mustard seed in a foot bath helps relieve respiratory congestion. For the foot bath mix one-tablespoon ground mustard seed with 2 quarts hot water. Mustard greens are a good source of beta-carotenes, calcium, and iron, as well as vitamin C.

Oregano

In Jamaica, oregano incense is used to help prevent and soothe coughs and other respiratory complaints. In ancient Greece oregano tea was used to treat poisonous insect bites, coughs and digestive problems. It is an excellent digestive aid.

Parsley

A breath freshener as far back as the early Romans, parsley is considered a herbal multivitamin. A cup of minced fresh parsley (about 4 oz, or 100g) contains more beta carotene than a large carrot, almost twice as much vitamin C as an orange, more calcium than a cup of milk, and twenty times as much iron as a serving of liver. It is a mild diuretic, and can stimulate menstruation. Chinese and German herbologists recommend parsley tea to help control high blood pressure, and Cherokee Indians use it as a tonic to strengthen the bladder. To make parsley tea, steep two teaspoons of bruised fresh parsley leaves in one cup of boiling water, covered, 10 minutes. Strain and take 3 times a day for water retention.

Peppermint

This herb is extremely popular in the Middle East, as a tea, condiment, and candy. In ancient Greece it was used to freshen baths, to treat hiccups, and soldiers rubbed their weapons with it for good luck. In the Middle Ages it was recommended for digestive distress; merchants sprinkled it around grain and cheeses to keep rats away. Monks used it to polish their teeth with fresh peppermint leaves for a brighter smile. The menthol helps soothe stomach lining, fend off nausea and vomiting, and encourages digestion by stimulating the gallbladder and liver, especially after a fatty meal. It can help relieve flu symptoms and clears congestion from the head. French bicycle racers drink a combination of peppermint and rosemary tea before racing. Peppermint tea creates a cooling sensation on the skin, so it's good for menopausal women. Too much peppermint tea may inhibit iron absorption in anaemic people.

Rosemary

In ancient Greece, rosemary was credited with having positive effects on the mind, and students tucked fresh rosemary sprigs in their hair when studying, to help them remember better. It has been a popular folk cure for stress and to ward off the evil eye. Rosemary contains a compound called rosmaricine that seems to relieve headaches the same way aspirin does, but without irritating the stomach; it can also soothe the digestive system. It's extremely high in calcium, a mineral known to calm the nerves: one tablespoon of dried rosemary contains about 42 mg.

Sage

Native Americans use sage for "smudging" ceremonies to clean areas of bad feelings and negative emotions. The sage is tied into bundles, called "smudge sticks", and lit, so they produce silvery smoke, and then waved around rooms, offices, houses, cars, or wherever else they're wanted. The Latin name for sage is "salvia", which means "salvation". Ancient Arabic and Chinese herbalists believed that drinking sage tea enhanced mental and spiritual clarity.

Modern herbalists report that sage's camphor, tannin, and other components have antiseptic properties. It can help treat sore gums and mouth ulcers. To make a mouthwash, steep one teaspoon of fresh sage or ½ a teaspoon dried in one cup of hot water, covered, for 4 minutes. Add a ¼ teaspoon salt and ½ teaspoon cider vinegar or lemon juice. Swish around mouth to help ulcers, or use as gargle for sore throat, but do not swallow. Sage tea can help prevent blood clots from forming, and is useful in the prevention and treatment of heart attacks. However, it also can cause uterine contractions, so pregnant women should avoid it. Use very small amounts to flavour stews and soups.

Tarragon

An excellent breath freshener, which takes care of the garlicky or oniony smells. It also creates a slight sensation of numbness in the mouth, and was given by Arab physicians as a precursor to bad-tasting medicines. Tarragon contains rutin, which is being investigated as a cancer cure. As it is high in potassium, it can help regulate blood pressure levels. Use fresh in salads, not as tea, or dried in sauces and stews—always moderately, as it is quite strong.

Thyme

This herb goes back to Biblical times, and in Greece lambs were made to graze on fields of wild thyme to make their meat tastier. A Middle Eastern variety is called *zatar*, which is used abundantly in cured olives, spinach pies, grilled vegetables, and herbed breads. Thyme contains a volatile oil, thymol, with antiseptic and antibacterial properties. It helps keep mouths and gums healthy, and helps heal coughs and is often used in commercial mouthwashes and commercial cough syrups. Thyme tea is excellent for fighting chest colds: steep 2 tablespoons fresh or 1 tablespoon dried thyme in boiling water for 4 minutes. Five drops of essential oil of thyme in ½ cup olive or grape seed oil makes a fine massage oil, good to combat coughs, sore throats, colds, and cranky digestion. Massage into chest, throat, feet, or back.

■ ■

3. Foods That Can Make Us More Intelligent

Brain Facts

The human brain weighs about 1.4 kilograms. It is about 2% of the total body weight but uses about 20% of the oxygen used by the entire body while at rest. Most of the brain cells are present from birth and so the increase in weight comes mainly from growth of these cells. During the first six years of a person's life he learns and acquires new behaviour patterns at the fastest rate in life. A network of blood vessels supplies the brain with the vast quantities of oxygen and food that it requires to keep functioning.

Brain Food

In recent years a lot of research has gone into finding that can keep the brain cells working at optimum level. The market is flooded with packages designed to provide food to promote intelligence.

Research has proved that certain kind of foods play a very significant role in improving memory and keeping the brain cells active.

The food that we eat everyday has a massive influence on the functioning of the brain and keeping it fit for performance. Elements like diet with low nutrients, exposure to the environmental toxins in our everyday living, stress, working round the clock against the dictates of our body clock, constant intake of stimulants like alcohol, tobacco, caffeine and junk foods to keep us going, all have an enormous affect on our mental functions.

The brain is constantly active, receiving information from the senses about conditions both inside the body and outside it. It is burdened with the enormous task of rapidly analysing all the information and sending out messages that control body functions and actions.

Memory And The Brain

As we age, we tend to lose some of our memory, eventually leading to a senile stage. It need not be so. One can retain a grasp over mental faculties with a little effort. Like any organ, the brain needs to be constantly exercised and kept in use.

Memory is the ability to remember something that has been learned or experienced. It is a vital part of the learning process.

Memory and the loss of it is a complex process. Time has a lot to do with memory. It is easier to remember things from the recent past than those which took place long ago.

Brain Fatigue

The brain is the largest consumer of the energy that our body produces. To process information efficiently, to access important data, to store necessary information, it needs oxygen, glucose and other nutrients. Lack of these leads to short-term memory loss and mental fatigue.

Memory loss occurs due to a lot of reasons. Although it primarily happens due to ageing, stress too can lead to forgetfulness. Clinical factors can also take their toll on the brain. Certain medications have side effects on the brain and cause fogginess and lack of concentration. Nutrition can affect the brain's working. The kind of food you eat can aggravate your mental inefficiencies. Thus it is very important to maintain a healthy food diet including all the nutrients necessary for proper functioning of the brain.

The Food Factor

Just like every organ in the body, the brain needs to be fed. If it doesn't get a constant supply of glucose for energy, it lets us know; symptoms of sluggishness, lethargy, dizziness and even fainting can occur.

Free radicals generated by the body could lead to erosion in the functioning of the brain. Waste products released by the body when we burn food for energy production is the free radical phenomenon. These free radicals can often lead to some loss of memory over the years.

What Are Free Radicals?

Free radicals and antioxidants are two words that we increasingly hear in the context of health and ageing. Let us get a clear picture about antioxidants and free radicals.

In a perfect world, energy is balanced and synergy abounds. The same idea applies to health when our bodies are fit and in chemical balance. But today's world is far from perfect. Our lives are typically stressful and we consume toxins on a daily basis, which ultimately alter our delicate biochemistry and wreak havoc on our internal chemical reactions. Compromised immune systems and increased exposure to free radicals eventually wear us down, ageing us prematurely, or bringing on fearful diseases like cancer. But powerful natural compounds called antioxidants form a front line of defence that attack and neutralize hordes of free radicals, helping us restore our health and live longer, happier lives.

A freshly cut apple will turn brown in a matter of minutes. Iron, when exposed to water and air, starts to rust. These chemical changes are the result of oxidation, the process by which a compound reacts with oxygen. Oxidation in the body creates free radicals in the fats, tissues, and bloodstream. The higher the number of free radicals, the greater the level of oxidative stress.

Oxygen is a critical element in the water we drink and the air that we breathe—without it we would not survive. Yet normal cellular reactions create toxic forms of oxygen that are free radicals such as super oxide, hydroxyl and lipid peroxides, singlet oxygen, and hydrogen peroxide. Small amounts of free radicals in the body are a good thing - too many, however, accelerate ageing and disease.

Not all free radicals are bad. Free radicals produced by the immune system destroy viruses and bacteria. Others are involved in producing vital hormones and activating enzymes that are needed for life. But most of us are bombarded by a multitude of environmental toxins like smog, cigarette smoke, heavy metals, gasoline derivatives, ultraviolet radiation, and other carcinogenic chemicals that are also sources of free radicals. A healthy body can normally keep its free radicals in check, but if the immune system is weakened or the free radical load is too high, cellular damage results.

A significant cause of ageing is cellular free radical damage. As we get older, an increased amount of free radical garbage accumulates in our bodies. The good thing is that we are not completely powerless. Antioxidant supplements can help protect us from the damage of free radical bombardment.

How Antioxidants Work

Antioxidants are compounds that neutralize free radicals by giving them the necessary electrons they crave. Antioxidants can be vitamins, minerals, hormones, or enzymes. Although a certain amount is manufactured in the body as enzymes or hormones, most of our antioxidants come from fruits and vegetables.

Although many antioxidants can be obtained from food sources, it is difficult to get enough of them to hold back the free radicals constantly being generated in our polluted environment.

Certain antioxidants protect specific parts of the body against certain kinds of free radicals. For example, vitamin E protects the fats in cell membranes. In addition to fighting free radicals, antioxidants stimulate the immune system, reduce inflammation and fever, and help control pain. Once an antioxidant has neutralized a free radical, it is essentially "spent".

Maintaining a healthy immune system, reducing stress, and consuming antioxidants can minimize free radical damage. Conditions that can be avoided or improved using antioxidant therapy include cancer, coronary heart disease, autoimmune disorders, rheumatoid arthritis, cataracts, diabetes, menopause, fertility, and neurological disorders such as Alzheimer's disease and Parkinson's disease.

Antioxidant Sources

Vitamin C

Probably the most well-known antioxidant, vitamin C helps minimize free radical damage to the neurological system. It also protects other antioxidants in the body, such as vitamin E. In addition to neutralizing free radicals, vitamin C detoxifies the body, reduces high blood pressure, lowers cholesterol, and fights cancer.

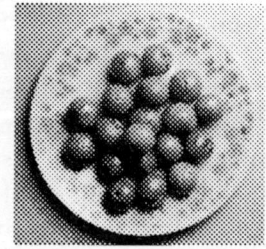

It has the beneficial effect on glutathione levels and helps prevent free radical damage to the brain cells. In the presence of high levels of glutathione, the body's immune system functions efficiently and prevents damage to the brain cells.

Vitamin A and Beta-carotene

Both vitamin A and beta-carotene are powerful free-radical scavengers that help the skin, mucous membranes, circulatory system, and cholesterol levels. In particular, beta-carotene is very effective in neutralizing the single oxygen-free radical.

More than 600 different types of carotene have been identified from fruits and vegetables, only a few of which have been studied. Preliminary research indicates that alpha-carotene is up to 100 times more powerful as an antioxidant than beta-carotene. Others include lutein, gamma-carotene, zeaxanthin, and lycopene, a known cancer fighter that occurs in high concentrations in tomato products.

Vitamin E

This antioxidant prevents the oxidation of lipids (fats) in cell membranes, which strengthens the outer cell layers against free radical attack. Vitamin E works best in the presence of selenium, another antioxidant, and helps protect vitamin A. Vitamin E stimulates the immune system, improves the circulatory system and oxygen absorption, fights cancer, and has a role in preventing cataracts.

Vitamin E helps protect the brain against oxidative stress. An intake of about 400 mg every day can be very helpful.

Chocolates

People with a sweet tooth need no longer feel guilty each time they pop a chocolate into their mouth. Scientist recently discovered that chocolate contains phenolics, an antioxidant believed to reduce overall chances of contracting heart disease. Pure chocolate may be the best chocolate around. That's because the fat in pure chocolate usually comes from cocoa butter, which has a high content of stearic acid, the saturated fat that doesn't hurt blood cholesterol level.

What's better, white or dark chocolate? Generally, dark chocolate is made from a higher content of cocoa butter and also contains many phenolics. White chocolate usually doesn't have very many phenolics, but is loaded with cocoa butter. A dark chocolate bar is considered the most beneficial, followed by fudge syrup, baking chocolate, chocolate fondue, and semisweet chips.

Coffee

Brewed coffee seems to create hundreds of new chemicals that appear to have antioxidant qualities. Each chemical is present only in tiny amounts, but taken together in a cup of coffee they could add up to have about the same antioxidant effect as three oranges.

Selenium

Selenium has been found beneficial in the fight against free radicals. It is found in the highest concentrations in seafoods, grains, muscle meats, and Brazil nuts. A multi-vitamin that contains between 70-100 mcg is recommended, but an additional supplement is not necessary. Selenium can also help prevent cancer.

Zinc

Just like it protects your car from rust, zinc has antioxidant properties that protect the body. Zinc is required to maintain effective levels of vitamins E and A. It is also a key ingredient in the very important antioxidant enzyme called superoxide dismutase (SOD).

Pycnogenol

It is an effective antioxidant. Common sources are the bark of the French maritime pine tree (Pycnogenol), grape seed, lemon tree bark, peanuts, and cranberries. Research indicates that this compound may be 20-50 times more potent than vitamins C and E. Besides, it keeps joints and skin supple, promoting a youthful appearance. It also strengthens capillaries, improves circulation, reduces joint pain, and protects nerve tissue.

Other Plant Sources

Several popular supplements like bilberry, ginkgo biloba, and garlic are very strong antioxidants. Bilberry helps eliminate free radicals from capillary walls and red blood cells; it is also known to control arthritis. And its ability to improve vision was first observed during World War II when it was discovered that British pilots, who ate bilberry jam, had excellent twilight vision.

What Really is Brain Food?

Once free radicals have been taken care of, the brain automatically functions better. The other items food elements that can be called brain food are :

- Vitamin B12 : Helps in improving concentration and memory. As we grow older the body is unable to absorb enough B12 from food. This leads to neurological disturbances like loss of balance, muscle weakness, poor vision and mood disturbance. If the deficiency over a period of time, it can precipitate pseudo-senility, a condition that hampers memory retention. Taking a supplement of Vitamin B12 can reverse the condition. The good sources of this vitamin are milk and milk products, meat, eggs, fish and most non-vegetarian foods. Vegetarians have to resort to Vitamin B12 supplements to protect the brain from the effects of ageing.

- Vitamin B 6 : Found in banana, wheatgerm, pulses, brown rice and brewer's yeast. Promotes clear thinking.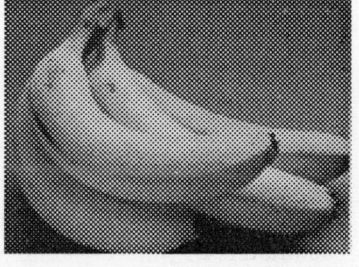

- Nuts like almonds, walnuts, sesame seeds, soybeans, whole wheat and wheat germ, pumpkin seeds, lecithin and choline activate the brain and improve its performance.

- Citrus fruits, fresh fruits and carrots keep the brain alert.

- Choline, lecithin, egg yolk and soya bean, improve concentration and memory retention.

Smart Ways to Feed Your Brain

Fatigue and a decline in mental alertness are the result of inadequate nutrients and oxygen in the brain, and lead to a decrease in brain function. Additionally, free radical damage causes diminished neurological function. If you're feeling groggy and foggy, supplements can help. The neurons in the brain require delivery of nutrients and oxygen, as well as removal of waste.

As we age circulation can be compromised to varying degrees. Certain supplements can boost circulation to ensure the adequate delivery of nutrients and oxygen. Ageing presents another problem: healthy brain function is related to flexible cell membranes, which allow the smooth flow and exchange of information. As the brain ages, cell membranes become rigid, hampering the flow of information.

Environmental factors and the rigours of everyday life present a big problem in the form of free radical damage. Free radicals are unstable chemicals formed in the body during normal metabolic processes and from exposure to external sources of toxins like cigarette smoke and air pollution. Even though they're a part of the body's natural chemistry, free radicals can damage cells if they exist at higher levels than normal.

Because free radicals are particularly attracted to fat cells, the brain with its relatively high fat content is especially vulnerable to free radical damage. Antioxidants help stop the progress of free radicals before they can attack healthy cells. In theory, a well-balanced diet should supply adequate amounts of antioxidants.

In reality, because of excess stress on the body and brain, environmental pollution and a reliance on processed foods, most people don't get enough antioxidants. For the ultimate brain protection, supplemental forms of antioxidants are advisable. Adequate nutrition is a major consideration for mental function. The brain is a relatively small organ, but a hungry one: it typically eats up about a quarter of the energy produced by the body. As such, it's highly susceptible to nutrient deficiencies.

At the minimum, it must receive adequate nutrients to allow the synthesis and release of neurotransmitters. Mom's stories about brain food do have a basis in fact: fish, for example, is packed with compounds that help promote optimal mental functioning. The problem is, the most concentrated sources of brain nutrients are found in foods that most people have reduced or eliminated from their daily diets, like red meats, organ meats and eggs. But as awareness of the brain's nutritional needs grows, so do the number of supplements in the market.

A plethora of products that promise alertness and increased mental health function are available. Most work by either increasing circulation to the brain, providing nutrients for energy, or protecting the brain against the ravages of ageing. Some work by providing an instant boost through short-term stimulants.

Brahmi *(Bacopa monniera)*

Brahmi was traditionally used to treat mental illness including epilepsy. It can help strengthen memory, elevate brain function, increase concentration and mental focus, enhance mood and reduce the effects of stress. In India, it has long been incorporated in hair oils for massage. It has been used to provide a cooling effect to the scalp and to relax the nerves.

Brahmi contains substances called bacosides, which are responsible for improving memory and memory-related functions by enhancing the efficiency of nerve impulse transmission. Bacosides work by repairing damage to worn-out neurons.

Flower Essences

Flower therapy is a method of treating various psychological and emotional imbalances to prevent their manifestation as physical illness. Flower therapies may be helpful in treating various types of mental disorders, including anxiety, depression and stress. One study on flower essences showed that flower therapy was effective in nearly 90 percent of subjects. Flower essences are thought to work by encouraging a more balanced emotional and mental state.

Bilberry

Long known for its ability to improve eyesight, bilberry can help brain function as well. By increasing circulation and blood flow, bilberry works in much the same way as ginkgo. Additionally, it's a potent antioxidant and can prevent free radical damage to the brain.

Gotu Kola

It is regarded as the most widely used herb in Indian ayurvedic medicine. Traditionally used as a nerve tonic and a general tonic in times of physical and mental exertion, it is also widely used to assist in pain relief of arthritis. In ayurveda, the herb is also used for ailments of the nerves and mind including epilepsy, schizophrenia and memory loss. The Chinese value Gotu Kola more as a plant that increases longevity and brain capacity than for any other purpose.

It is able to rebuild energy reserves and for this reason it is called 'food for the brain'. It increases mental and physical power. It combats stress and improves reflexes. Gotu Kola has an energising effect on the cells of the brain and is also said to help prevent nervous breakdown. It can relieve high blood pressure, mental fatigue and senility and helps the body defend itself against various toxins. It contains vitamins A, G, and K and is high in magnesium.

Some sources indicate that massive doses of Gotu Kola can produce narcotic effects. The evidence for this effect and Gotu Kola is considered to be quite safe by nearly all herbalists.

B Vitamins

There are many other natural substances that can help feed the brain and optimise its function. For instance, the B vitamins are crucial enzymes for the metabolism of the glucose that gets translated into energy.

In the mid-1940s and 1950s, scientific research clearly showed that healthy brain functioning depends on sufficient amounts of B vitamins. Experts still tout the importance of B vitamins, particularly the following five (these vitamins are all water-soluble and should be taken together for maximum benefit) :

B1 (thiamine) helps convert glucose into energy. Thiamine supplementation also appears to elevate mood. In a study, 120 young women were given either placebo or 50 mg thiamine daily for two months. Before-and-after tests were conducted to assess their mood, memory and reaction times.

-The women who took the thiamine supplements reported feeling significantly more clearheaded, composed and energetic than the ones who were on a placebo.

B3 (niacin) enhances the ability of red blood cells to carry oxygen. It is also vital to the formation and maintenance of many tissues, including nerve tissue. A severe niacin deficiency produces pellagra, a disease characterized by the three Ds: dermatitis, diarrhoea and dementia.

B6 (pyridoxine) is needed for the production of amino acid-derived neurotransmitters such as norepinephrine, serotonin and dopamine. B6 deficiency can cause many ailments including slow learning and visual disturbances. Low levels of this vitamin may also provoke epileptic seizures in people prone to them.

B12 (cobalamin) plays an important role in the formation of the myelin sheath around nerve fibres. It also helps the body transport and store folic acid. Vitamin B12 deficiency can cause pernicious anaemia, nerve dysfunction (weakness, poor reflexes and strange sensations in the arms and legs) and impaired mental activity. It has also been linked to depression, especially in the elderly.

Folic acid is necessary for DNA synthesis; it plays an essential role in all cell divisions and the development of the foetal nervous system. As many as 31 to 35 percent of all depressed patients have folic acid deficiencies

The B vitamins are also important for the reactions which power synthesis of our brain neurotransmitters, chemical signals that the brain uses to carry out physiological functions. B vitamins are needed for the synthesis of the neurotransmitters dopamine, norepinephrine and serotonin. Dopamine and serotonin are especially related to feelings of contentedness, well-being and satiety (fullness). Low levels of serotonin are associated with depression, anxiety and cravings.

Siberian Ginseng

This is another quality herb beneficial to the brain and the central nervous system. It is known as an "adaptogen" and serves to balance the internal organs. It has consistently demonstrated an ability to increase the sense of well-being in a variety of psychological disturbances, including depression, insomnia, hypochondriasis and various neuroses.

Ginseng not only has powerful antioxidant properties, it also has been found to increase circulation which is associated with improved oxygen delivery and increased energy, similar to the effects of ginkgo biloba.

St. John's Wort

This is a herb that is rapidly becoming popular for its effects on mood and anxiety. Recent research indicates that St. John's wort may be acting by increasing levels of the "feel good" neurotransmitter called serotonin, which actually is "brain food". St. John's wort has been effectively used to control depression.

Fish Really is Brain Food

The value of fish was recognised long before scientific medicine proved the point. For centuries it has been seen as "brain food" and from the 1650s people have been taking cod liver oil to fight bone disease and aches and pains. Medical research has begun to confirm some of old physicians' practices and old wives' tales. More recent studies have suggested that fish oil reduces the chances of heart problems, helps prevent hyperactivity in children, is useful in treating depression, lowers aggression under stress and eases pain from arthritis. The role fish oils may play in fighting cancer, especially breast cancer, is also under investigation.

Oily fish like salmon, kippers and tuna are especially beneficial. The importance of the oils lies not only in the protein, vitamin A (good for vision, hair, eyes and nails) vitamin D (good for teeth and bones) and trace elements such as phosphorus and iodine, but in the large supplies of polyunsaturated fatty acids known as omega-3. This seems to help protect against heart disease by lowering levels of plasma triglyceride, which is associated with high cholesterol.

If you're a woman looking to reduce your risk of stroke, think of fish as a good thing. The more fish women eat, the greater the benefit, says a new study. Studies found that women who ate fish just one to three times a month had a 7 percent lower risk of stroke than those who ate it only once a month. Increasing the fish intake to once a week could result in stroke risk going down by 22 percent. Two to four times a week reduces risk to 27 percent, and eating fish five times a week or more brings down the risk of stroke by up to 52 percent.

Experts say the likely reason fish protects women is the concentration of omega-3 fatty acids, nutrients that prevent the formation of clots, mostly by making blood less "sticky". This, in turn, reduces the risk of ischaemic stroke, which is caused by blood clots that form either in the brain (leading to a thrombotic stroke) or elsewhere in the body and then travel to the brain (causing an embolic stroke). Another study found that omega-3 fatty acids reduced platelet clumping by up to 11 percent.

The study also found that the benefits of fish oil might be increased if the overall diet is also low in fat.

Omega-3 fatty acids protect the heart in several ways. By preventing the heart from beating too fast, they guard against the formation of blood clots and also prevent the build-up of plaque in the heart arteries.

Prevents High Blood Pressure

Eating fish regularly with omega 3 polyunsaturated fatty acids is said to significantly lower blood pressure in people suffering from hypertension. According to a group of doctors from John Hopkins Medical School, USA, 3 grams or more per day of fish oil (6-10 capsules) can lead to reduction in the blood pressure in hypertensive individuals, lowering systolic pressure by an average of 5.5 mm Hg and diastolic pressure by 3.5 mm Hg. It is more effective in individuals who have really high blood pressure.

Prevents Cancer Too

Including fish in your diet may even prevent certain types of cancer. Although in-conclusive in humans, studies in animals have found that some fish fats, rich in omega-3 fatty acids, suppress cancer formation.

It's important to note that not all fish are alike. Light-meat fish, like flounder or whiting, have only about 0.5 grams of omega-3 fatty acid per 4-ounce serving, while dark-meat fish, such as salmon, sardines, mackerel or bluefish, have roughly 1.5 grams of the protective fatty acid in the same amount of fish.

If you're going to eat only one serving of fish a week, experts recommend choosing a dark-meat fish.

Although consumption of fish was said to aid in reducing the risk of sudden death, it did not seem to change drastically with the increase in consumption. In other words, although eating fish once a week seemed to work, eating it more often did not work better.

Fruits and Vegetables are also Brain Food

We have always assumed that eating fruits and vegetables was good for health because they were good sources of a wide variety of vitamins (vitamin C in citrus fruit, vitamin A in carrots, folic acid in greens). Then, it became important to eat fruits and vegetables because they were good sources of fibre. 100 grams of apple for example contains 2.7 g of fibre while 100 grams of turnip contains 2.0 g of fibre. Fruits and vegetables also contain antioxidants and it is the effects of these dietary sources of antioxidants on brain that have an anti-ageing effect.

The brain is a strange organ. Firstly, it is not as dynamic as other organs in the body–the turnover of cells in the brain is almost zero, unlike the liver or the lungs. This means that the brain is particularly sensitive to damage because once the brain cells are injured or killed they aren't replaced. Secondly, it contains low concentrations of antioxidants without which the brain tissue is vulnerable to damage.

The relation between antioxidant damage to the brain and the onset of Alzheimer's disease and Parkinson's disease has not been proven as yet, but there have been some indications that there is a link.

The phytochemicals in spinach and strawberry extract, particularly those with antioxidant properties, could provide protection against the onset of these degenerative diseases. However, experiments to prove their efficacy are difficult to carry out. Foods such as spinach and strawberry extract may be more effective than just pure vitamin E because foods and extracts contain a cocktail of phytochemicals rather than just one active ingredient. A mixed diet with plenty of fresh fruits and vegetables is still probably the best dietary advice anyone can follow.

Memory Food

In a study of elderly people, the participants who consumed the most fruits and vegetables and the least fat and cholesterol performed best on cognitive capacity tests. This is probably because fruits and vegetables are an excellent source of antioxidants.

Blueberries and blackberries, in particular, are packed with brain-protecting antioxidants. Other nutrient-rich sources of antioxidants include prunes, raisins, garlic, kale, raw spinach, tomatoes and dried apricots.

Finally, if you're trying to ward off mental decline, a moderate amount of alcohol may be helpful, as long as you are not predisposed to addiction. A study of elderly people revealed that low to moderate alcohol consumption, about one drink per day, appears to protect against failing memory. Almost 30 percent of your daily calories feed your brain, so it's no wonder that food has such a great impact on the strength of your mind.

■ ■

4. Foods That Elevate Our Moods

After extensive research in the last two decades, scientists have finally confirmed the link between food and mood. Although food choices may depend on taste or other conscious criteria, there is evidence that people often make unconscious food choices that change the chemistry in the brain, putting them in a better mood. These foods serve as anti-depressants. Chronic depression has also been linked to a long-term subtle deficiency of certain nutrients that presumably go unnoticed by the body.

Improve your Mood with Food

Foods seem to manipulate mood by effecting serotonin, one of the brain's most remarkable neurotransmitters. Eating foods that lead to abnormal amounts of serotonin in the nervous system can make people depressed. On the other hand, foods that lead to normal amounts of serotonin in the brain elevate moods more or less the same way, as do drugs.

In our century, depression strikes at an earlier age. Could diets be the cause? Some researchers suspect that we eat too little omega-3 fats, found especially in fatty fish like salmon, herring, and mackerel. One type of omega-3 fat, DHA, makes up 30% of certain brain cell membranes in healthy people.

A study showned that there was a definite link between depression and omega-3 fats. It was found that the more severe the depression, the lower the level of omega-3 fats. Now a new study has compared levels of omega-3 fats in healthy people and people diagnosed with depression. This study revealed that the levels of omega-3s were 40% lower in patients with depression, on an average.

Salmon can Make you Smile

Is salmon nature's Prozac? It isn't known yet whether depression causes lower omega-3 levels. Possibly it's vice versa. But one theory is that diets deficient in omega-3s make you more vulnerable to depressive tendencies. If you have other risk factors, low omega-3s could tip you over the edge.

A single serving of 85 gms of salmon contains almost 2 grams of omega-3 fats, about ten times the average intake. Eating fish rich in omega-3 fats, like salmon, just might help us fend off serious blues. Besides salmon, other choices include canned white tuna, mackerel, sardines, herring or anchovies.

Vitamin D can Cure the Blues

Do you get depressed as the days get shorter? In fact, the weather has a lot to do with our mood. Sun is a vital source of cheer. You must have experienced a dull and depressive mood on cloudy days when the sun is not visible. If you are one of those who feel depressed in the absence of the vital sunrays, Vitamin D may be the answer to your problem.

In a small study, college students who took 400 IU of vitamin D during the winter reported feeling more enthusiastic, inspired, and alert than those who took a placebo. How could vitamin D fight depression? Some experts think it may affect levels of the mood-lifting brain chemical serotonin.

The Candy Connection

Some researchers suggest that people can eat certain types of foods, such as sweets and carbohydrates, to alter their frame of mind as well as to provide comfort. Dr. Judith Wurtman, USA, in her research study, found that eating certain 'mood' foods could have a significant impact on a person's state of mind. The results indicated that the sugar and starch in carbohydrate-loaded foods boost the brain chemical, serotonin, which is important in governing mood.

"When people are stressed because of work, family affairs, PMS (premenstrual syndrome), winter darkness, they feel a need to eat carbohydrates," says Dr. Judith Wurtman. Her research also shows that certain foods high in serotonin, such as high-fat sweets, can produce cravings for comfort. Wurtman's research additionally suggests that carbohydrate-rich foods, such as breads, cereals, pasta, fruit and starchy vegetables elevate serotonin levels, which helps people feel more relaxed and calm. Low serotonin level is linked with increased aggression and depression.

In addition to food's suggested mood enhancing properties, Wurtman's research shows that high protein foods, such as cottage cheese, yoghurt or milk, beans, peas, nuts and soy products, release other substances that increase alertness and allow people to react and think more quickly.

Mood can also be affected by high carbohydrate intake, Wurtman said. She found that when people consume enough carbohydrates - between 35 and 40 grams - on an empty stomach, they had the edge taken off their mood and felt better.

Chocolates for Mood Elevation

Chocolate has also been labelled as one of the most powerful mood elevators. It is full of mood-enhancing chemicals. To start with, it is loaded with sugar, which is a carbohydrate and triggers the release of seratonin. Chocolate also contains fat, which in itself provides a feeling of satisfaction since it answers the urge for calories. Chocolate is also said to have the same mood-enhancing chemical that is found in marijuana, although in much smaller quantities.

To test the theory that chocolate enhances mood, a study was conducted at the University of Pennsylvania. Students who felt the urge to eat chocolate were given either:

1. Milk chocolate,
2. White chocolate (which contains no cocoa, just cocoa butter and flavouring); or
3. Pills containing stimulants found in chocolate.

The findings were quite interesting. The pill didn't do the trick, but both the white and milk chocolates did satisfy the students. The results suggest that it is not some secret chemical ingredient in chocolate that provides the euphoria, but the sensory experience, the taste, the smoothness and the aroma. Perhaps the mood-enhancing chemicals are just the "icing on the cake."

Dealing with Depression

A link between food and mood can be traced to neurotransmitter activity in the brain. **Complex carbohydrates** as well as certain food components such as **folate** (folic acid), **magnesium, niacin, omega-3 fatty acids, selenium**, and **tryptophan** may decrease symptoms of depression.

What you should Eat and Why?

Complex carbohydrates

Consuming foods that are high in tryptophan along with foods high in complex carbohydrates will help enhance the proper absorption of tryptophan more effectively. Carbohydrates may also boost the serotonin activity in the brain. Foods that are often referred to as "comfort foods" tend to be high in complex carbohydrates.

Leading food sources of complex carbohydrates are brown rice, potatoes, white rice, beans and wheat.

Folic acid

Because folic acid is often deficient in people who are depressed, getting more of this vitamin through foods may help. The vitamin appears to have the ability to reduce the high levels of homocysteine associated with depression. Leading Food Sources of folic acid include asparagus, beets, broccoli, Brussels, avocados, spinach, cabbage, bok choy, beans, chickpeas, soyabean, lentils, oranges, peas, turkey.

Magnesium

Magnesium is a mineral that may ease symptoms of depression by acting as a muscle relaxant. Leading food sources of magnesium are spinach, avocados, almonds, buckwheat, amaranth, chocolate, pumpkin seeds, oysters, sunflower seeds, Brazil nuts, Quinoa and barley.

Niacin

Based on niacin's well-recognized role in promoting sound nerve cell function, some experts recommend this B vitamin for relieving depression as well as feelings of anxiety and panic. Most B-vitamin complexes contain niacin in sufficient amounts for this purpose; they also offer the mood-enhancing benefits of other B vitamins. Leading food sources of niacin are brown rice, lamb, pomegranates, tuna fish, wheat, turkey and chicken.

Omega-3 fatty acids

Certain omega-3 fatty acids may be beneficial for depression. Docosa hexaenoic acid (DHA) is the building block of human brain tissue. Low levels of DHA have been associated with depression. Leading food sources of omega-3 fatty acids include walnuts, salmon, trout and tuna.

Honey and lemon balm

Honey contains laevulose, dextrose and other sugars, which give instant energy and a person feels active and stimulated after its ingestion. An excellent brain tonic is to soak seven almonds in water overnight and after removing the skin, taking them with a tablespoon of honey in the morning.

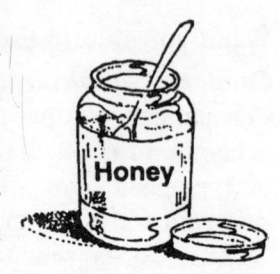

Lemon balm is an important culinary herb of the mint family. It is considered an antidepressant, and has been used successfully in the treatment of mental depression. It alleviates brain fatigue, lifts depression and raises one's spirits. A cold infusion of the balm is reputed to be excellent for its calming influence on the nerves. To make the infusion, soak about 30 grams of it in half a litre of cold water for twelve hours. The infusion is then strained, and taken in small doses throughout the day.

Selenium foods

There is interesting new evidence that eating foods rich in the trace-mineral selenium can improve moods. In a controlled study, 50 healthy men and women, aged 14 to 74, took either 100 micrograms of selenium a day or medicine for five weeks or a placebo. After six months, they switched to the opposite pill. The selenium in their diet was also measured. Throughout, tests were conducted to judge their moods as to whether they were more composed or anxious, agreeable or hostile, elated or depressed, confident or unsure, energetic or tired and clear-headed or confused. The surprising results were that moods improved markedly when the subjects got enough selenium.

The researchers concluded that a subtle selenium deficiency, not enough to cause a disease, puts a curb on mood. Thus, correcting the slight deficiency would normalise the mood, but getting more of the mineral would not boost it further. Rich vegetarian sources of selenium are garlic, onions, tomatoes and milk. It is believed that selenium influences mood presumably due to its antioxidant power.

Foods That De-Stress

Stress is the bane of today's society and plays havoc on our physical and mental makeup. Psychological stress activates the adrenal glands to discharge stress hormones called cortisol, which help us survive the stress but are harmful to our health. When a person is exposed to prolonged periods of stress, he can develop ailments like high blood pressure, stomach ulcers, cancer and various immune disorders such as rheumatoid arthritis, depression etc.

Food has a profound effect on both mind and body. Health is a reflection of our physical, mental, emotional and spiritual well being. A person with a disturbed mind cannot have a healthy body because the mind is the monitor of our physical health. Research at the National Institutes of Health in the USA has been looking at how stress affects the mind and body. One of the scientists, Dr. Pamela Peeke, focussed her work on the relationship between stress and weight gain. It was found that people who are stressed-out often turn to food for solace, and eat more than normal. Dr. Peeke found that the stress released fat accumulation can begin in people as young as 20.

Stress is one of the largest killers of mankind, today. It is the cause of most of our illnesses, whether physical or mental. Stress has a very negative impact on our digestive system. The body can assimilate the nutrients from food only when the mind is in a relaxed condition. No matter what you eat, if the mind is disturbed, your body will not gain any benefits from the nutritive components of your food.

There are, however, a few foods that help the body cope with the demands made by stress. When the body is under stress the demand for nutrients is more as key nutrients are burned up faster. In order to derive the maximum benefits from a nourishing diet, one needs to follow three essential steps–

- Eat under a stress-free and pleasant atmosphere.

- Eat just enough to repress hunger; overeating can be hazardous. Overload the digestive system by overeating and it will make you lethargic, sleepy and inactive.
- In case you suffer from excessive stress, eat foods that counteract stress.

Foods that Counteract Stress

During stress, the body needs more of certain nutrients because they are burned up faster than usual. Stress increases the demand for vitamin C, Vitamin A, Vitamin B-complex, proteins, magnesium, antioxidants and essential oils. To counteract the stress effects, one needs more of these nutrients.

There is a high concentration of vitamin C in our brain tissues, more than any other tissue in the body. Vitamin C is a powerful antioxidant, that is used up quickly during stressful periods. One needs to cater to the high demand for this vitamin during high levels of stress. An amount between 500-1,000 milligrams would be required to combat the stress after-effects. The best sources of vitamin C are citrus fruits like oranges, potatoes, tomatoes, and leafy green vegetables.

Vitamin A is another requirement during times of stress. It is needed for maintenance of skin, mucous membranes, bones, teeth and hair, eyesight, and reproduction. Vitamin A may also protect against cancer. Liver (especially fish liver), egg yolk, fortified margarine, oily fish, oranges, apricots, carrots, tomatoes, melons, and dark green leafy vegetables contain this vitamin in abundance.

Magnesium is found in dark green leafy vegetables, nuts, seeds, whole grain foods, legumes, milk.

Proteins are of two types - animal protein and vegetable protein. Animal protein can be found in foods like meat, fish, egg and all dairy products, while vegetable protein is found in grains, beans, pulses, nuts, seeds and sprouted seeds.

Stress increases the generation of free radicals in the body, which are the main cause of cancer. The only elements that can fight free radicals are antioxidants, found in plenty in cruciferous vegetables like cabbage, cauliflower, broccoli etc. They are rich in bio-flavinoids, which are powerful antioxidants. During stressful times, the body generates a whole lot of free radicals, which cause harm to the body cells. Bio-flavinoids protect the body against cell damage caused by free radicals.

Another important source of antioxidants is green tea. It contains an abundance of polyphenols which are active agents protecting against heart disease and cancer. The polyphenols also protect against the damages caused by stress. Chamomile tea is a powerful anti-stress agent. It relaxes and soothes the mind and promotes sound sleep.

Fruits are an essential ingredient, which could provide the required amounts of antioxidants required to counteract stress. They contain simple sugars and complex carbohydrates, which help raise the seroton levels in the bloodstream. Serotons are the 'feel good' neurotransmitters, which elevate mood and fight depression.

Vegetable and fruit juices are also a good source of antioxidants. A regular glass of any fruit juice or vegetable juice can go a long way in helping the body cope with the detrimental effects of stress.

■ ■

5. Unhealthy Food

In different parts of the world, over hundreds of years, people's bodies have adapted to a variety of diets. But the alterations in diet have been so rapid that the body has been unable to adjust fast enough. For example, the intake of sugar has increased manifold over the past few decades. The consumption of fats, food additives, soft drinks, refined and processed foods have increased to unhealthy proportions. Most good value foods have been replaced by fast foods. Eating out is another trend that is neither healthy nor economical.

Most people heap their systems with unhealthy food, which causes a lot of harm. Some of the damaging food habits become so addicting that people do not like giving them up or settling for something "insipid" like vegetable juice.

Sugar

Sugar is the quickest energy-giver, and easy on the digestive system. It passes almost at once into the blood stream, and gives us a feeling of 'immediate lift'. This works mostly when we choose foods naturally high in sugar, like fruits, dry fruits, milk and certain vegetables (peas, carrots, sweet corn, sweet potato etc.). Besides providing quick energy, other essential nutrients from these foods help maintain our pep and good looks.

However, dependence on concentrated sweets and soft drinks for quick energy, especially in between meals, definitely works against our health and appearance.

Sugar is a source of 'empty' calories since it yields 100% energy and no other nutrients. Those who derive a large chunk of their energy from concentrated sugary food are likely to be poorly nourished. This is because these foods are eaten at the expense of other more nutritious foods thereby depleting the amount of vitamins, minerals and protein in the body. Overweight is also encouraged by a sweet tooth since excess sugar is stored as body fat that we don't need.

Sugar per se does not cause heart disease, diabetes or any other problems. However, excess consumption does lead to fat, which in turn leads to diabetes and heart disease. Dental caries (cavities) are definitely encouraged with high-sugar intake. Cavities are formed when bacteria that live on the teeth metabolise sugars to acid, which dissolve the enamel and the underlying structure. Gastric distress and overfullness in the stomach occurs when sugar is eaten in large amounts at one time. This, along with quick energy release, dulls the appetite for the next meal.

Some researchers have suggested that sugar affects behaviour, especially in children. They claim that sugar creates an excited even antisocial state, which may lead to violence and disruptive behaviour. But most researchers find that sugar in itself is not the villain, it is probably the excitement or tension in situations where high-sugar foods are prevalent such as parties and festive occasions that is the culprit.

Sugar is neither good nor bad if eaten in moderation. By regularly visiting the dentist, practising good dental hygiene, following a good balanced diet plan while keeping weight under control, consuming sugar in reasonable amounts poses no health threats. What should be a desirable level of sugar intake? Less than 10-15% of total kilocalorie intake should be quite adequate because this allows for 10-15 teaspoons (present in foods and added) on a 2,000 kilocalorie diet.

The desirable way to consume sugar is through the diet as it occurs naturally in fruits, fruit juices, vegetables, cereals, breads, dry fruits, milk/milk products, since they also contain other vital nutrients. Cut down on sweets, candies, soft drinks, chocolates, ice creams, and sweet biscuits. The amount of sugar eaten in the day should be distributed among three meals, rather than consumed in a large amount at one meal or as a snack. Also gradually reduce the sugar in foods prepared at home by one-third. Try new recipes. Use home prepared items (with less sugar) instead of commercially prepared ones that are higher in sugar. Experiment with such spices as cardamom, cinnamon, nutmeg, and saffron to enhance the flavour of foods. Have cereal, milk and fresh fruits with little or no sugar added. Cut down on the amount of sugar used in tea or coffee. Avoid pre-sweetened cereals, milk, canned fruits, soft drinks and fruit juices, sweet biscuits and other baked items. Reach for fruits or dry fruits instead of concentrated sweets for dessert or a snack since they provide valuable nutrients along with fruit sugar.

The time and place to eat a concentrated sweet is as a dessert after a good balanced meal. You have then eaten the vegetables, fruits, cereals, pulses, milk, and meat and already got your supply of 'protective' vitamins, minerals, protein and fibre. When planning a meal, keep in mind the dessert lest you add unneeded calories that end up as body fat. If you plan ahead, a sweet will give you a feeling of completeness and enjoyment as a climax to a meal without those terrible pangs of guilt.

Refined sugar supplies only 'empty' calories, i.e. no nutrients, only energy. It is the major cause of tooth decay and it is a principal factor in diabetes, obesity, and certain other disorders. It makes us hungry by creating a 'roller coaster' effect in our blood sugar levels: blood sugar soars, the pancreas reacts by secreting more insulin, then levels rapidly plummet, making us tired, hungry and depressed. This is the low blood sugar syndrome, hypoglycaemia.

Refined sugar passes quickly into the blood stream and shocks the stomach and pancreas. It causes an acidic condition in the body and the body rushes to neutralize this using its reserves of minerals. Calcium is one of these and is used up quickly. Calcium is one of the essential nutrients used in the contraction of muscle fibres. A muscle cannot relax without proper amounts of calcium.

Over time, conditions of hypoglycaemia and diabetes can result from constant intake of sugar. The adrenal glands also become stressed, resulting in fatigue and impaired immune function. Sugar contributes to arteriosclerosis, anxiety, irritability, shakiness, headaches, insomnia and many more symptoms and conditions.

Caffeine

It is actually a drug and is addictive. Caffeine produces an initial surge of energy, alertness, and well-being through its direct effect on the nervous system and adrenal glands. With this constant stimulation the nervous system and adrenal glands become stressed and overworked causing fatigue and immune system problems in the long run. This stimulant also activates the contraction of muscles adding to tightness that may already be there.

Coffee and caffeine-rich foods, like chocolate, tea, and cola drinks, produce   a release of the body's stored sugar to combat the influx of what is essentially a poison. Like alcohol it provokes hypertension and nervous symptoms. Cholesterol levels go up and B vitamins and some minerals are depleted. Excess caffeine may also be involved in breast and prostate problems.

Coffee beans are the major source of caffeine. They are grown with the use of pesticides and herbicides that are toxic in nature. Caffeine is also found in chocolate, colas and other soft drinks and some over-the-counter drugs such as Excedrin and Anacin. Some signs of caffeine problems are fatigue, headache, depression, insomnia, anxiety, muscle tightness, high blood pressure and PMS.

People suffering from insomnia will realise that their sleep improves after stopping that coffee before bedtime. Coffee and tea are known to stimulate gastric secretion. Patients with peptic ulcer should restrict their use. They should drink fewer cups and add more milk or cream to their beverage. Heart patients and those with high blood pressure should also avoid or reduce the frequency and strength of their drink because caffeine stimulates cardiac muscles, increases the cardiac output and has a deleterious effect on blood vessels.

Cerebral vessels are constricted by caffeine. There is a risk of an increase in blood pressure if tea or coffee is taken in excess. Expectant mothers and those breast-feeding should cut down on their coffee. The caffeine in the coffee drunk by the mother is ingested by the foetus in the womb and by the suckling child through breast milk. The infant has no means of breaking down the components of the same and accumulates it in the body. Drinking of coffee is also harmful to the pancreas and may lead to pancreatic cancer.

Drinking Coffee Raises Blood Pressure

Did you Know?
1. Caffeine produces transient hypertension in men at risk for hypertension.
2. Caffeine further raises blood pressure in men who are already hypertensive.
3. While caffeine increases the blood pressure of normal men, the increase is not clinically significant.

The Study

These conclusions were drawn after a study conducted by scientists who examined the immediate effects of caffeine on arterial blood pressure (BP) in 182 men at risk for hypertension. There were five groups, classified on the basis of resting BP:
1. Men with optimal BP
2. Men with normal BP
3. Men with high-normal BP
4. Men with stage 1 hypertension
5. Men with confirmed hypertension

BP was measured after 20 minutes of rest, and again 45-60 minutes after the oral administration of about 250 mg of caffeine.

The Findings Were

1. Caffeine raised both systolic and diastolic BP in all five groups of men.
2. For both systolic and diastolic BP, the greatest increase in BP was observed in men with confirmed hypertension, followed by those with stage 1 hypertension and high-normal BP, followed by those with normal and optimal BP.
3. The caffeine-induced increase in BP was 150% greater in diagnosed hypertensives than in those with optimal BP.
4. Before the administration of caffeine, 78% of diagnosed hypertensive men and 4% of stage 1 men were hypertensive. After caffeine ingestion, 19% of the high-normal men, 15% of the stage 1 men, and 89% of the diagnosed hypertensive men had BP in the hypertensive range.

5. All men in the optimal and normal groups remained in the normal BP range.

Comments

1. The average cup of coffee contains about 150 mg of caffeine. The dose of caffeine administered in this study, therefore, was a little less than that contained in two cups.
2. The clinical significance of this transient caffeine-induced rise in BP is uncertain. For instance, there are no data to suggest that the risk of coronary or cerebrovascular disease events is raised shortly after the consumption of coffee.
3. While caffeine raises blood pressure, it also dilates peripheral blood vessels, including those of the heart. Thus, a negative effect is offset by a positive effect.

Recommendations

1. A guarded recommendation may be made that hypertensive men should cut down on caffeine intake.
2. A more confident recommendation may be made that patients should not drink caffeine-containing beverages (such as coffee and cola drinks) before a medical examination during which BP will be recorded.

If you get a headache when you don't have your morning coffee, you are addicted to this drug. Gradually ending the intake of this substance is recommended. Begin with cutting back on the daily amount and substitute with other products such as teas and coffee substitutes.

Caffeine Levels

The caffeine content of a cup of coffee depends on the type of bean and how it was processed and brewed. Tea's caffeine content increases the longer it steeps.

Item	Caffeine (mg)
Coffee (1 cup)	
Regular, drip	60-180
Regular, percolated	40-170
Regular, instant	30-120
Decaffeinated, brewed	2-5
Decaffeinated, instant	1-5
Tea (1 Cup)	
Brewed	25-110
Instant	25-50
Cola drinks and chocolate	
Cola drinks (1 bottle)	30-60
Chocolate milk (250 ml)	2-7
Cocoa (1 cup)	2-20

Soft Drinks

Soft drinks are bad for health due to the same caffeine factor and sugar content.

Eliminate the intake of soft drinks substituting with water and lemon or herbal teas. Drinking synthetic cold drinks has become a fad. These contain gas and synthetic colours that may look very attractive, but contain toxic substances. Carbon dioxide is a gas we breathe out. Through these cold drinks, we are ingesting this gas and our body will have to spend some energy in expelling it.

Animal Protein

Although animal flesh, eggs and dairy produce provide the complete protein necessary for health, in excess it can be harmful. People who live on a high animal protein diet are thought to be more disposed to bowel cancer, hypertension, diverticulosis and atherosclerosis.

Animal fats are saturated fats and bring about free radical formation to some extent. They not only enhance ageing but also hasten the onset of diseases like cancer of the colon and breast. Most popular sources of animal fats like cheese, full fat milk, ghee, red meat, beef and skin of chicken can cause a lot of damage to one's health.

Excessive intake of red meat also stimulates calcium loss, and reduces bone density leading to osteoporosis. Instead, eating white meat like chicken and turkey is better than eating red meat. However, do not eat the skin of chicken since it has high fat content.

The animal protein component in food should be cut down, especially as one grows older. It is a misconception that only non-vegetarian food provides complete protein. Vegetarian foods can also provide all the protein elements when they are properly combined. In fact, more and more people are turning to vegetarianism because of the benefits it provides.

Refined Foods

The inevitable result of a diet high in refined starches is a decrease in the consumption of fibre. Without fibre, food can take up to 70-80 hours to pass through the digestive tract. Lack of fibre in the diet is responsible for sluggish bowels, constipation and more serious disorders such as diverticulosis and possible cancer of the colon. A whole food diet, with plenty of fresh vegetables and fruits, provides sufficient fibre.

Saturated Fats

Excess saturated fats have been implicated in cancers, obesity, cardiac disease, and a host of other disorders. Too much saturated fat makes too much cholesterol, which may build up on the arterial walls, from childhood, resulting in atherosclerosis (hardened arteries from fatty deposits). All the fried food that goes under the label of gourmet food and attracts hordes of eager diners to high-flying restaurants helps the consumption of an unhealthy amount of saturated fats. Bland food, which has less of oil and spices, is hardly palatable to the adventurous tongue and so people flock to the eateries that cater to the rich and spicy favourites. The result is an increased intake of fats.

Dairy products and fatty meats are major culprits; wild game has more polyunsaturated fat, and contains a substance that is thought to protect against atherosclerosis.

Food Preservatives and Additives

Unless you grow all your food in your own garden and prepare all your meals from scratch, it's almost impossible to eat food without preservatives added by manufacturers during processing. Without such preservatives, food safety problems would get out of hand, to say nothing of the grocery bills. Bread would get mouldy, and salad oil would go rancid before it's used up. Food law says preservatives must be listed by their common or usual names on ingredient labels of all foods that contain them — which is most processed food. You'll see calcium propionate on most bread labels, di-sodium EDTA on canned kidney beans, just to name a few. Even snack foods — dried fruit and potato chips contain sulphur-based preservatives. Manufacturers add preservatives mostly to prevent spoilage during the time it takes to transport foods over long distances to stores and then our kitchens. Rapid transport systems and ideal storage conditions help keep foods fresh and nutritionally stable. But breads, cooking oils, and other foods, including the complex, high-quality convenience products consumers and food services have come to expect usually need some kind of preservative to keep them going.

Preservatives serve as either anti-microbials or antioxidants — or both. As anti-microbials, they prevent the growth of moulds, yeasts and bacteria. As antioxidants, they keep foods from becoming rancid, browning, or developing black spots. Rancid foods may not make you sick, but they smell and taste bad. Antioxidants suppress the reaction that occurs when foods combine with oxygen in the presence of light, heat, and some metals. Antioxidants also minimize the damage to some essential amino acids—the building blocks of proteins—and the loss of some vitamins.

Since most people don't have access to farm fresh food all of the time, many people rely on processed items as part of their daily sustenance. Food additives help maintain the freshness and shelf life of such food products because without them, they would spoil quickly due to exposure to air, moisture, bacteria, or mould. Either natural or synthetic substances may be added to avoid or delay these problems.

Food additives may be used in a variety of ways, including:

- To maintain consistency or texture — to sustain smoothness or prevent the food from separating, caking, or clumping.
- To improve or retain nutritional value: Enrichment replaces nutrients lost in processing — this occurs with grains, as some vitamins and minerals are lost in the milling process. Fortification adds a nutrient that wasn't there before and may be lacking in many people's diets. Iodised salt is an example. This has proven useful in preventing goitre, a thyroid disease caused by a deficiency in iodine. Enriched and fortified foods are labelled as such.
- To delay spoilage.
- To enhance flavour, texture, or colour.

Since ancient times, salt has been used to cure meats and fish, and sugar has been added to fruits to preserve them. Herbs, spices, and vinegar have also served as preservatives.

Food additives don't always connote something "bad." For example, ascorbic acid refers to vitamin C and alpha-tocopherol is actually vitamin E.

Some uses and examples of food additives are:

Antioxidants

Prevent spoilage, flavour changes, and loss of colour caused by exposure to air. Vitamin C and Vitamin E are used as antioxidants e.g. ascorbic acid in butter.

Emulsifiers

Used to keep water and oil mixed together. Lecithin, for example, is used in margarine, baked goods, and ice-cream. Mono- and di-glycerides are other elements found in similar foods and peanut butter. Polysorbate 60 and 80 are used in coffee lighteners and artificial whipped cream.

Thickening Agents

Absorb water in foods and keep the mixture of oil, water, acids, and solids blended properly. Alginate is derived from seaweed and is used to maintain the texture in ice cream, cheese, and yoghurt. Casein, a milk protein, is used in ice cream, sherbet, and coffee creamers.

Colours

Make food more colourful; two examples are tartrazine and sunset yellow.

Flavour Enhancers

Bring out flavours in food; a well-known one is monosodium glutamate (MSG).

Anti-caking Agents

Stop powdery foods from forming lumps, as in salt.

Nitrates

Act as a preservative in many foods but may be added to foods, such as pork, to give a pink colour.

Are Additives Safe?

The vast majority of additives and preservatives appear to be safe. They have been tested by many laboratories throughout the world before being used in foods. However, individuals may be "sensitive" to various additives and preservatives. Government agencies are supposed to control what substances, and in which amounts, may be used in the production of food.

Who do They Affect?

In the majority of cases, individuals with some form of allergy, e.g. asthma, hay fever, urticaria, etc., will be affected by these substances. A few additives and preservatives can affect non-allergic people. Some of these substances cause more reactions than others. For example, reactions to sulphur dioxide and sodium benzoate occur more commonly in asthmatics than reactions to the colorant tartrazine.

What Kinds of Reactions can Occur?

The reactions to food additives are not the kind of allergies as one sees with an egg allergy, but usually a type of chemical reaction. Reactions depend on the type of preservative or additive ingested. These may include vomiting, rashes, hives, a tight chest, headaches, worsening of eczema, and many other symptoms.

Are there other substances that these reactions may be confused with?

Similar reactions may occur with an allergy to a food such as egg, nuts, etc. Some foods have natural chemicals that may affect you too. For example, fish that's not fresh may have a high level of histamine, cheese may have tyramine, and you may react to the histamine in wine and not the sulphur dioxide!

Which Additives result in Side Effects?

It is not possible to cover all the additives and preservatives that may result in reactions, but these are some of the more important ones.

Preservatives: Sulphur dioxide and sodium benzoate often cause "tight chests" in individuals who have asthma. Many people also complain of a scratchy feeling at the back of their throats. Although these are the common reactions, others such as rashes may also occur. Sulphur dioxide may be labelled as sodium metabisulphite, potassium metabisulphite, sodium or potassium bisulphite, or sulphite.

Some foods that may contain sulphur dioxide are:
- Some fruit juices,
- Concentrated soft drinks,
- Dried fruit,
- Wine, beer,
- Some sauces,
- Pickles,
- Hamburger patties

Some foods that may contain sodium benzoate include:
- Fruit juices,
- Soft drinks,
- Foods with fruit.

Flavour enhancers: The most famous is monosodium glutamate, commonly called MSG. Eating foods with this additive may result in tight chests in asthmatics. This reaction may occur immediately or 6 to 12 hours later. A condition called "Chinese Restaurant Syndrome" may occur in any individual. This reaction can occur about 20 minutes after a food containing MSG is eaten on an empty stomach. Typical symptoms include headache, a burning sensation along the back of the neck, chest tightness or pain, nausea, sweating and a sensation of facial pressure. "Pins and needles" or tingling may be experienced in the limbs or face and head. It is not a common condition.

Some foods that may contain MSG are: Oriental food, packet soups, sauces, soya sauce, seasoning. MSG is also thought to occur naturally in mushrooms and tomatoes.

Antioxidants: These are substances that prevent oily foods from becoming rancid. Some individuals complain of reactions to butylated hydroxyanisole (BHA) or butylated hydroxytoluene (BHT). Fortunately, reactions to these substances are not common. Reactions include rashes, hives, and occasionally "tight" chests.

Colourants: Colourants may be natural or synthetic. Reactions, although not common, can occur to both types. The best-known colourant is tartrazine. Tartrazine is an azo dye, so if you react to this colourant, you should avoid all of the azo dyes. Although many people are concerned that they may be affected by colourants, not many individuals are in fact affected. Thus not all asthmatics need to avoid tartrazine. Whether tartrazine or other colourants can result in hyperactivity in children is still controversial.

Some foods that may contain colourants include:
- Fruit juices
- Soft drinks
- Sweets
- Desserts
- Toppings
- Syrups
- Cooking oils
- Sauces, and
- Pickles

Sweeteners: The artificial sweetener aspartame may cause rashes or hives in sensitive individuals. This sweetener is added to many "low calorie" foods.

Salicylates: Found in aspirin, acetyl salicylic acid may result in a "tight" chest or hives in some asthmatics. A different form of salicylic acid can be found in a variety of spices and foods. Some health professionals believe that this form can result in many side effects, including hyperactivity in children.

Some foods that may contain salicylic acid include:

- Ice cream
- Curry powder
- Paprika
- Dried thyme
- Berries
- Ginger
- Almonds
- Apricot
- Oranges
- Tea, and
- Honey

How do I know whether I am affected?

This may not always be obvious. In some instances, the reaction will immediately follow the ingestion of an additive or preservative, as with sulphur dioxide and sodium benzoate. In other cases, the reaction may be delayed for 6 to 24 hours.

What can I do to see if I am affected?

You may have to keep a diary and record all the food you eat, the time it was eaten, and when the reaction occurred. You will then need to see if there is a pattern to the reaction. Unfortunately, there is no blood or skin test available to check whether you are affected. Your doctor may suggest a "challenge" with the substance to see if you are indeed affected.

5 Key Points to Remember:

1. Preservatives and additives cause chemical and not allergy reactions.
2. Only some asthmatics will react to these substances.
3. There are no reliable tests to confirm sensitivity to these chemicals.
4. Keep a diary of what you eat and when reactions occur, to look for a pattern.
5. Read all food and ingredient labels carefully

Eggs

Eggs have been held responsible for the increase of cholesterol in the body. Too many eggs can be quite harmful but if one removes the yolk, the harmful effect can be controlled to a large extent. The benefits are that an egg is a rich source of nutrients so it should not be completely cut out of the diet. Restricting the intake to about 4-5 per week should work fine and if the yolk is removed, the number could go up to 7 per week.

The egg yolk is rich in freely emulsified, easily digestible fats. Carotenoid pigments make the yolk yellow in colour. It contains proteins and is rich in fat-soluble vitamins as well as minerals like phosphorus, calcium and iron. The composition of a duck's egg and a hen's egg is similar. An average egg contains 100 mg of cholesterol and that is what makes it dangerous for middle-aged people.

Egg and Diseases

- Allergy – Egg is a common allergen in infants, children and adults, producing articaria and asthma. In all allergic patients care should be exercised not only to avoid egg, but also with regard to eatables made out of egg e.g. cakes and biscuits.
- Atherosclerosis – Fats in egg yolk contain saturated fatty acids. The fact whether eating one to two eggs per day raises blood cholesterol and predisposes a normal individual to heart disease is still under extensive research.
- Gall bladder disease – Fats in eggs causes contraction of gall bladder and this may produce pain and discomfort if the gall bladder is diseased. Such patients should avoid eating eggs.
- Egg-borne infections – As the shell of an egg is porous, it is not always sterile. When eggs are laid on dirty, marshy land, micro-organisms penetrate the shell. The most common infections are caused by the salmonella group of organisms, giving rise to typhoid fever and gastro-enteritis. However, if eggs are cooked well, these diseases can be prevented.

Fat Facts
What are Fats?

Fats that we eat are made up of two chemicals: fatty acid and glycerol. These are formed from carbon, hydrogen and oxygen.

These can be either saturated or unsaturated depending on the structure of the fatty acids. The more hydrogen atoms a fatty acid has, the more saturated it is. The degree of fatty acid saturation varies widely.

How does the Body use Fats?

Fats are part of the wall surrounding every body cell. Fats in small amounts are essential and perform some pretty vital jobs. They insulate the body against cold, serve as a reserve store of energy, act as shock absorbers around the bones and organs, insulate nerve cables, lubricate the skin and help transport certain essential vitamins.

Harmful Effects of Fat

The excess fat is stored in body cells making you overweight. By consuming fats/oils that are easily oxidisable, you predispose your body to the risk of free radical formation. These free radicals make the body cells diseased and dysfunctional. Besides the medical repercussions such as stroke and heart ailments this excess fat also accelerates ageing. The type of fat you take in is the key to how fast you age.

Which Kind of Fat is Good?

Cholesterol rich foods such as egg, red meat, butter and cheese are oxidised easily and promote premature ageing. This type of fats ruins the arteries by elevating the bad cholesterol or the low-density level (LDL) cholesterol. They oxidise the LDL cholesterol, which can then penetrate the artery walls thereby clogging them and increasing the possibility of heart attack. On the other hand, mono-unsaturated fats are slow to oxidise and hence don't cause cell damage. They include olive oil, almond oil, walnut oil, fish oils, flaxseed oil, etc.

Animal fats like butter and ghee increase the production of inflammatory agents in the body causing arthritis, choking of arteries, migraine and some skin problems. All these are also considered the manifestations of ageing.

The Right Choice

- Switch to olive oil
- Use olive oil for cooking and as salad dressings. Research

has shown that consuming at least two tablespoons of olive oil can cut the risk of breast cancer by about 30 percent. Moreover, like the other mono-unsaturates, it also selectively lowers the LDLs leaving the (good) HDLs intact

- Use minimum quantity of other oils
- Using 2-3 tsp. of other oils daily is just enough for the necessary body function.

Cooking with Oils

Corn Oil

Although corn oil is healthy, this is the least satisfactory of the recommended vegetable oils for cooking purposes. For salads, the flavour is rather powerful. If you do not find the flavour attractive, try mixing in some olive oil for cooking or salads.

Olive Oil

This is delicious and can be used for everything, but it is expensive. It has a lovely fruity flavour, which varies tremendously from country to country. However, it is wasteful to use this oil for frying, since it loses its delicious flavour at high temperatures. Use it for rubbing on to meat or fish before grilling, for marinades, for lubricating freshly cooked pasta and, of course, for all salads.

Salad Oil

Mixing four tablespoons of sunflower oil with two dessertspoons of walnut oil, which has a delicious flavour, makes an interesting salad oil.

Soya Oil

This is good for frying, but it starts to taste and smell a bit strong at high temperatures. It has the right consistency for salads. This is the oil used in Japan, where they have so little heart disease. Nutritionally, it is a highly recommended oil.

Sunflower Oil

This oil is excellent for frying as it is almost tasteless and does not smell. It gives a very crisp result. As it is so light and thin it makes a rather dull salad dressing. It is the most versatile of the recommended poly-unsaturated oils but it is expensive.

Say 'No' to Hydrogenated Oils

Never use hydrogenated oils because they increase the risk of heart disease and also produce more free radicals in the body, which in turn advance ageing.

Salt

Common table salt, known chemically as sodium chloride, is the main source of sodium in our diets. Sodium is an essential nutrient required by the body to help regulate its fluid balance, maintain heart rhythm, conduct nerve impulses, and contract muscles. For body requirement, a safe minimum is 500 milligrams of sodium, about a quarter teaspoon of table salt is enough. Most people consume about twice the daily maximum (3000 milligram of sodium – about teaspoon and a half of table salt) recommended by doctors.

The common belief is that blood pressure rises with age. Expected blood pressure is usually expressed as "100 plus your age". This holds true for many individuals but it is not normal. In fact, blood pressure does not rise with age in everyone, although a large proportion of people – 15% of young adults and 40% of elderly – have high blood pressure.

In certain societies blood pressure does not rise with age and hypertension does not occur. These societies include Pacific Islanders, South American Indians and Aboriginal tribes people. And there are others, all of whom live in harmony with their natural environment. They eat a variety of vegetables and fruits and freshly prepared, unsalted food, so the amount of sodium in their diet is a small proportion of what we eat. This is an important difference, which could account for the differences in blood pressure between them and us.

Reduction of sodium intake to 1 millimole per kilogram of ideal body weight will lower blood pressure in those with hypertension. In others, it will prevent hypertension from too much sodium. If sodium intake is reduced while people are young, the rise in blood pressure with age could be prevented.

The relationship between salt intake and hypertension (high blood pressure) is complex and not fully understood but the direct relationship between sodium consumption and the high incidence of high blood pressure has been demonstrated in a number of studies.

About 10-15 percent of people are actually 'sodium-sensitive'; meaning that consuming too much salt directly elevates their blood pressure.

Healthy adults should reduce their sodium intake to no more than 2400 milligrams per day. This is about 1¼ teaspoons of sodium chloride (salt). To illustrate, the following are sources of sodium in the diet.

¼ teaspoon salt	=	500 mg sodium
½ teaspoon salt	=	1,000 mg sodium
¾ teaspoon salt	=	1,500 mg sodium
1 teaspoon salt	=	2,000 mg sodium
1 teaspoon baking soda	=	1,000 mg sodium

Where is the Sodium in the Foods We Eat?

There are two major sources of sodium in the foods we eat. It is present in raw foods but the major source is sodium which is added. This occurs during manufacture and preparation of food. Additional amounts in the form of sodium chloride may be in sauces and flavouring agents.

What is a Normal Sodium Requirement?

The amount of sodium required will depend on ideal body weight and is equivalent to 1 mmol per kilogram, per day. A man who, for example, is 176 cm tall and weighs 70 kg is at an ideal body weight. Therefore, his recommended dietary sodium intake is 70 mmol of sodium per day. Ten mmols (millimoles) or meq (milli-equivalents) of sodium is contained in 0.58 grams of sodium chloride. Sodium makes up 40% of sodium chloride by weight.

Infants require less sodium (10-49 mmols a day) than adults. Sufficient sodium to meet a baby's needs is present in breast milk even though, when compared with cow's milk, breast milk has only one-third amount of sodium. Older children up to their teens will need a slightly higher sodium intake per body weight than adults but this will be obtained if food intake is adequate to maintain growth and ideal body weight.

Sources of Salt

There are many hidden sources of salt. One of the main sources of sodium in the diet is a group of staple items – bread, butter or

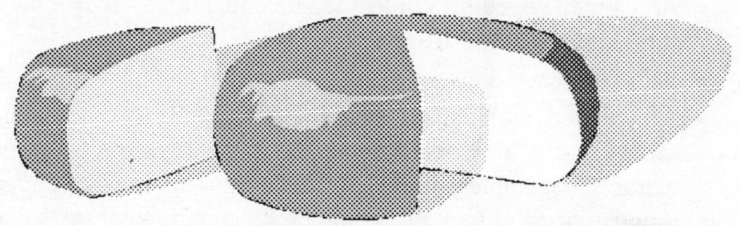

margarine and cheese. Breads generally contain salt and so do biscuits. Cheeses are very high in salt, too. Apart from these most of the processed foods like gravy powder, stock cubes, yeast extracts, peanut butter, pickles and olives also contain sodium.

Some minor sources of sodium in our diet are mineral replacement drinks, mega doses of vitamin C and some soluble painkillers.

The natural sodium content of fresh foods does not really present a problem because it is relatively low in most foods. Some seafoods are among the exception. Prawns and scallops, for example, have significant sodium content but these do not usually form a large part of most people's diet.

Protein foods from animal sources also have a relatively high content of sodium but, as the healthy diet pyramid indicates, we should all decrease our intake of animal products.

Milk, being an animal protein product, falls into this group and the recommended intake for an adult is 300 ml and, generally, this should not be exceeded.

High Sodium Items

- All canned, corned, and pickled meat or salted meat or fish. All processed meat e.g. corned beef, salami, chicken loaf, ham, bacon, sausages, Frankfurt, and tinned fish unless labelled no added salt.
- All hard cheese, especially Parmesan or Romano. Highly salted breakfast cereals, commercial cakes, pastries, buns, cake mixes. Take care with commercial dry biscuits and sweet biscuits, which can contain significant amounts of sodium.

- All canned vegetables unless labelled no added salt. Pickles, sauerkraut, minted frozen peas.
- All takeaway foods.
- All canned and packet soups, prepared sauces or sauce mixes, gravy powders, stock cubes, meat extracts, yeast extracts, vegetable salts, celery salt, garlic salt, lemon pepper, monosodium glutamate, commercial mayonnaise or salad dressings, commercial sauces, soy sauce, olives, salted nuts, snack foods e.g., potato crisps, meat and fish pastes, ordinary peanut butter.
- Milk chocolate, caramels, Dutch liquorice, fizzy lollies.

Alcohol

Like sugar, alcohol gives a false stimulus to the system and is rapidly followed by sedation and depression of certain body functions. It depletes the levels of vitamins, most notably the B and C group, and minerals, such as zinc, magnesium and potassium.

It is fashionable to imbibe alcohol and an increasing number of women are resorting to this practice although it has been found that the harmful effects of alcohol on women far exceeds those on men.

Eventually, alcohol takes a heavy toll on health, causing cirrhosis of the liver, gastric troubles, heart disease, muscle disorders, nervous system problems, sexual impotence, etc.

If natural fruit juices are kept warm for a few days and exposed to the air, the sugars in them will usually ferment to form alcohol. Starches, grains and potatoes can also be made to ferment. The alcohol we drink is called ethyl alcohol. Ordinary beers contain between 2½ and 4% of this alcohol by volume: 'special' strong beers may have as much as 8%. Wines generally range between 8-12%, and fortified wines (e.g. sherries and aperitifs) contain added spirits, which bring the alcohol content up to about 20%.

Social drinking within limits is not harmful but it is the problem of alcoholism, that can be hazardous.

What is Alcoholism?

Alcoholic drinks provide a source of energy for the body but contain relatively few nutrients and vitamins. Those who drink them moderately, in company, are 'social drinkers'. Some social drinkers become heavy drinkers, and may develop, without necessarily recognizing it, into excessive drinkers. These are people whose drinking leads to social, economic or medical problems. Alcoholism is a self-inflicted condition but its effects are not confined to the individual drinkers. It breaks up marriages, alienates children and loses people their jobs. Physically the effects can be disastrous. It is thought that around 70% of chronic alcoholics suffer from fatty infiltration of the liver and about 10% from cirrhosis of the liver.

Nutritional Values of Alcohol

Alcohol contains traces of vitamins and minerals, but its nutritional contribution to the diet is negligible. Beer, for example, is a relatively poor source of carbohydrates compared with fruit juice. And wine contains small amounts of niacin, riboflavin, iron, calcium, and potassium, but richer sources of these nutrients are found in foods.

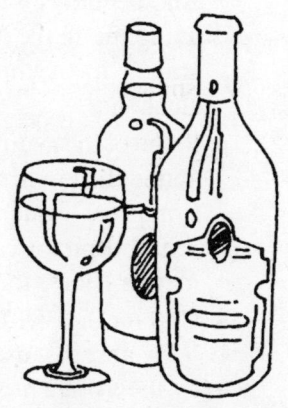

Because of its low nutritional content, alcohol is often described as providing 'empty' calories, but this doesn't mean they are few in number. Pure alcohol contains 7 calories per gram – fewer than fat but more than carbohydrates and protein. If you are trying to control your weight, consider that for the same 150 calories in a can of beer, you could eat a medium size baked potato, or 2 slices of whole grain bread.

Effects on Health

- Chronic heavy drinking is linked with an increased risk of cancer of the mouth, throat, oesophagus, liver, pancreas and rectum. The risk is heightened if a heavy drinker is also a smoker. Several studies have suggested that women who consume alcohol even moderately (as few as three drinks a week) have a higher risk of developing breast cancer than women who don't drink.

- Many alcoholics have peptic ulcers. Regular drinking causes chronic inflammation of the stomach, which in turn causes most alcoholics to lose interest in food. As a result of eating a small amount of convenience food, alcoholics often consume a diet low in vitamin content. They may nevertheless maintain a normal weight or increase in weight because alcohol substitutes for carbohydrates in the diet.

- Excessive alcohol may also **weaken the heart muscles,** causing the heart to enlarge and reducing the efficiency of the pumping action. Eating a balanced diet may protect a heavy drinker from some of these effects, but not all. Another effect is the nerve damage described as polyneuritis- a tingling in the hands and feet, and cramps in the legs, are among the symptoms – which may affect a fifth of all alcoholics.

- Some of the neurological complications, such as the 'shakes' and delirium tremens (hallucinations), are 'withdrawal symptoms', and alcoholics who have reached this stage need hospital treatment under special care. Others –severe memory loss, for example – may be permanent.

- Chronic heavy drinking has a serious impact on how the body absorbs, uses and stores food. Alcohol is metabolised by the liver, a process that takes precedence over other liver functions and interferes with that organ's effectiveness in processing nutrients. In a chronic heavy drinker, fat is stored in the liver instead of being metabolised efficiently. As a result, the liver grows larger and its ability to metabolise many vitamins and minerals is impaired. Damage to the pancreas, stomach, and gastrointestinal tract due to chronic heavy drinking may also hinder the absorption of nutrients.

- Vitamin and mineral deficiencies – particularly that of magnesium, calcium, phosphorus, zinc, pyridoxine, thiamine, riboflavin, niacin, folic acid and vitamins A, C and D – have been noted in alcoholics.

- Heavy drinking also leads to reduced dexterity. Alcohol is very rapidly absorbed and begins to act on the brain in about ten minutes. Co-ordination of hand and eye begins to fail, as does the ability to judge distance – precisely the brain function required to drive a motorcar or operate powered machinery safely.

Although these kinds of co-ordination fail – and sometimes brain damage can be permanent – verbal skill usually remains unaffected. So do not regard your ability to talk coherently as proof of your ability to drive safely. Drinking is also a major cause of accidents and violence both at work and home.

However, these physical and mental effects are complications of alcohol misuse and generally arise only years after the sufferer's personal, social and professional life has been destroyed. Care should be taken so that one does not reach that stage.

Fast Food and Junk Food

French fries, burgers, pizzas and the like are the hot favourite amongst the current generation. Exotic food is a symbol of prosperity and status.

` What is called fast food, or junk food, has very little to boast in the nutrition department. It caters more to the palate and satisfies the taste buds. Fast food is fashionable. The business enterprises that set the cash registers ringing in the west have now set their eyes on the Asian countries. The huge amounts set aside for publicity and advertising vouch for the target they have set for themselves. The convenience offered by readymade foods, home deliveries and fancy wrappings have caught the imagination of Indian consumers. It is so much more convenient to order for a pizza and sit back in front of the television, instead of slogging in the kitchen to prepare a wholesome meal. The trend of living on fast food or ready to prepare food is catching on in the developing countries at a rapid rate, much to the concern of health specialists.

Junk food needs to be junked without any thought, at the earliest. It is also a misconception that only western food is junk food. In fact, *pakoras, bhelpuri, kachori, chaat, samosa* etc. also fall under the same category, although the calories contained in them may not be as high as that in a hamburger or a pizza.

It is true that western junk food is rich in protein, since many of them – like hamburgers, rolls and hot dogs – contain a certain amount of fish, meat, chicken or bean component. They may even

117

provide some vitamins but what they supply in excess are factors that can be harmful. What are these harmful factors?

One thing they provide in plenty is calories. Whether it is the burger, the rolls, the pizza or the French fries, the number of calories they contain is enormous. Just one portion of a junk food item is enough to give calories required for the entire day. And if you take the help of some aerated soft drinks to gulp the fast food down, there are some more calories added to the kitty.

The worst part is that most of the calories come from fat. Ingredients like cheese, butter, mayonnaise and the deep-frying of most of the other elements add liberally to the fat content in the fast foods. The layer of cheese, mayonnaise and butter that goes into the pizza topping is bad news for the heart. And heaven help those of you trying to reduce weight. The other factor against deep-frying is that the oil is generally recycled. Everyone knows that recycled oil is carcinogenic so whether you are having *chaat,* burger with cutlets or samosa, the cancer factor is very active.

Sugar and sodium are some more of the hazardous elements that go in the preparation of junk foods. Sodium is just not salt. There are items which contain hidden sodium and they are equally bad. Some of the most popular stuff like popcorns, salted fries, chips and cheese have high sodium content. Even burgers, which contain salami, sausages and ham, have high sodium as well as fat content. The high level of sodium makes it hazardous to those suffering from hypertension. As for the sugar element, the soft drinks and ice creams are a major culprit. They account for excessive sugar content, which is harmful for diabetics. The caffeine content in the carbonated drinks is another health hazard. Caffeine interferes with the absorption of nutrients, robs the body of vitamin B, upsets the stomach and causes insomnia. Watch out before you gulp down the next cola, no matter what the advertisement says.

What is common in noodles, pizza, samosa, cakes, burgers and hot dogs? Foxed? They all contain refined flour, which has no fibre, whatsoever. Refined flour has nothing to recommend it. It is a big zero nutritionally with the additional ill effect of clogging up the intestines. So why settle for something that has nothing in it except a whole lot of calories?

And that is not the end of the subject. Most of the ingredients in the junk foods are canned, or bottled. The ketchup, for instance or the mayonnaise or the sausage, ham and salami contain food additives, which are known hazards and carcinogenic elements. Additives such as emulsifiers, antioxidants, stabilisers, anti-caking agents, preservatives and taste enhancers contain chemicals that cause numerous diseases. Apart from these elements, short shelf life, inadequate quality check, unhealthy cooking conditions and handling, all add to the hazardous nature of fast or junk food.

Let us just take a look at the two medium slices of pepperoni pizza you are consuming with great relish. The base is made of refined flour with food additives to make it rise. The calorie count is 640 kcal; apart from the calories, your pizza contains 36 gms of fat and 1,898 mg of sodium. It also contains other food additives that have been added to cheese to preserve and emulsify it. Hidden factors of sodium are also present in the ketchup along with some more food chemicals.

Want to top it up with some fries and soft drinks? Add 200 calories for the fries alone and the whole gamut of food additives, as well as sugar in the soft drink. Oh! I forgot to take the caffeine into account.

Do you still want to take your family out to the nearest pizza centre?

Dangers of 'Pan Masala/Gutka'

There is bad news for all those addicted to pan masala and gutka. Pan masala is a deadly combination of tobacco, highly processed betel nut and synthetic *katha*, besides lead, arsenic and magnesium carbonate. These substances cause oral cancer as their use brings about changes in the lining of the mouth and throat, weakening the layer of cells which give a protective covering and keep bacteria away.

The ill-effects of the regular consumption of pan masala and gutka on the human body has been accepted by medical experts worldwide. Eighteen to 20 per cent of cancers in India are of the mouth and throat, most the result of chewing of tobacco and consumption of pan masala and gutka.

Medical records show that 39.8 out of every one lakh men in Ahmedabad suffer from oral cancer, 33 in Bhopal, 25 in Mumbai, 23 in Chennai and 18 in the capital. The incidence of oral cancer among women is also increasing.

The countrywide data indicates that India is second to Brazil in the number of patients having mouth cancer. While in Brazil the main cause of such cancer is liquor consumption, in India it is mainly due to tobacco chewing.

Tata Institute of Fundamental Research, which screened over three lakh patients in different parts of the country, established beyond doubt that tobacco and betel nut chewing can lead to mouth and throat cancer.

This century has seen a global rise in tobacco-related cancers. Although tobacco chewing and smoking habits are recognized as risk factors for oro-pharyngeal cancer, chewing products such as pan masala and gutka continue to be introduced into the Indian market. The popularity of these products has ensured that tobacco-related cancers will continue to dominate the Indian scenario.

You could get leukoplakia, that is, white sores in the mouth that could lead to cancer. Your gums will recede or peel back, making you look distinctly awful. You will have bone loss around the teeth, adding to your dismal appearance. You could suffer from abrasion of teeth, that is, they could wear out, so that eating food could become torturous. Your tongue will become 'bald' so that eating hot or sour or spicy foods will become painful and difficult. But worst of all, you could get cancer. Studies have found high rates of leukoplakia (sores in the mouth) in smokeless tobacco users.

Food and Allergy

Which Foods Cause Allergic Reactions?

A few foods can trigger allergic reactions. Among the most common are cow's milk, eggs, wheat, soya, peanuts and fish. Allergic reactions to food may occur anywhere in the body, but usually in the digestive system, the skin, and occasionally in the nose and lungs - the places where the special immune system cells are stationed to fight off invaders that are inhaled, swallowed or come in contact with the skin. In most cases, foods cause reactions in allergy-prone individuals if they are swallowed. In certain people, food may cause reactions such as asthma if inhaled. For example, flour can cause asthma in bakers who are allergic to this substance.

How Common is Asthma in Persons with Food Allergy?

Food allergy is generally uncommon. It affects about 1% of children and 0.05% of adults (5 in 1,000). Skin symptoms such as eczema and hives and symptoms of the digestive tract such as stomach cramps, vomiting and diarrhoea are more common in food allergy than asthma. Asthma may develop in less than 5% of individuals who suffer from food allergy. In general, inhaled allergens such as house-dust mites, cat fur and pollen are more likely to trigger asthma than foodstuffs.

Diagnosis of Food Allergy

The diagnosis of food allergy is easy when the adverse reaction occurs soon after ingestion of an uncommonly used food item but is more difficult if the reaction occurs several hours or days later, or if a commonly used food is involved. In this situation a variety of diagnostic tests (skin prick test) can be used. At present there are no definite and reliable tests to diagnose food allergy. The final mainstay of diagnosis is the demonstration of the relief of symptoms on removal of a given food item and recurrence of symptoms on its re-introduction (eliminate-challenge testing).

How is Asthma Due to Food Allergy Treated?

The most effective approach to treating asthma related to food allergy is to avoid the offending food(s) in the first place. However, identifying the offending food may not be easy or it may not be possible to completely avoid it. In this situation, medication to control asthma must be taken by the patient. A number of new and effective medications are available to treat asthma and food allergy.

5 Key Points to Remember Regarding Food Allergy

- Food allergy is generally uncommon, affecting 1 in 100 children and 5 in 1,000 adults.
- Allergic reactions to food occur more commonly in the digestive system and the skin, and rarely in the lungs and nose.
- Asthma develops in less than 5 in 100 individuals with food allergy.
- Common foods causing allergy are cow's milk, eggs, wheat, soya, peanuts and fish.
- The most reliable way to diagnose food allergy is by elimination-challenge testing.

■ ■

6. The Anti-Ageing Food Plan

We all know that free radicals cause ageing so the wise thing to do would be to eat foods that maximize your antioxidant intake while minimizing your free radical load. This will actively resist the ageing factor.

You can easily achieve both goals provided you follow a low-fat, vegetarian diet—one in which the foods come only from plants, not animals. The anti-ageing food plan focuses on organically grown, unprocessed, chemical-free foods selected from the four food groups consisting of grains, legumes, fruits, and vegetables.

This diet is not only naturally low in fat but also naturally high in desirable complex carbohydrates. In fact, approximately 80 percent of the calories you consume in a day should come from complex carbohydrates such as whole-grain breads, cereals, pastas, brown rice, potatoes, yams, and squash. The other 20 percent of calories should come from protein and fat, in equal portions.

Eating this way automatically eliminates the free radical burden imposed by a high-fat diet. It also sidesteps other known toxins, including pesticides, food additives, alcoholic beverages, and sugar. By following this diet plan, you can protect your immune and cardiovascular systems from damage, prevent diseases of degeneration, and slow the ageing process.

By adhering to the diet plan, you accomplish two goals. First, you boost your intake of disease-fighting essential nutrients, antioxidants, phytochemicals, and fibre—the substances that reinforce your body's healing powers, increase its resistance to disease, and extend life span. Second, you sidestep disease-causing substances—the fats, sugar, white flour, pesticides, antibiotics, hormones, additives, and preservatives that undermine health and shorten life span.

Foods to Include

Before you begin the anti-ageing food plan, you have to make a commitment to stick with the diet that will substitute the meats, the dairy products, and highly refined and processed fare with the following foods:

Grains

What you need is a diet that is high in complex carbohydrates and low in protein and fat. So you'll be getting many of your daily calories from grains such as wheat, rye, oats (oatmeal and oat bran), millet, rice (brown, not white), and corn. For the most nutritional value, stick with organic, whole, minimally processed grains and grain products as much as possible.

Legumes

These are seed-pods—beans, peas, lentils, and the like. Stock your pantry with all-kinds: adzuki beans, anasazi beans, black beans, brown beans, chickpeas, green beans, green peas, kidney beans, lima beans, mung beans, navy beans, pinto beans, and, of course, soybeans and soy products (such as tofu, tempeh, and soy milk).

Fruits

You can't go wrong in this group, either—simply choose whatever is in season. Fresh fruits are preferable to frozen, since the freezing process can destroy some of the nutrients. As for juices, purchase organic products made from whole fruits or try making your own from organically grown whole fruits. Avoid juices made from concentrate as well as those with added sugar or with preservatives.

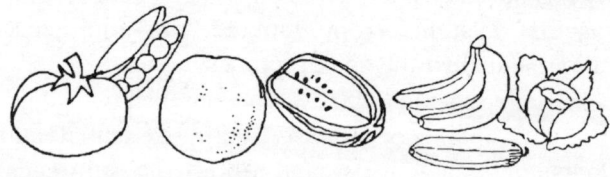

Vegetables

They are the most nutritious elements in an anti-ageing diet plan. They're also the best sources of protective phytochemicals. We are fortunate to have so many varieties of vegetables in our country. There is a whole range of green, yellow and red vegetables to choose from. No matter which ones you choose, you'll get bountiful amounts of vitamins, minerals, phytochemicals, and fibre. It is always a good idea to plan a menu which includes vegetables of all colours because that is the easiest way of ensuring that most of the vitamins and other essentials are available to you.

Beets, broccoli, Brussels sprouts, cabbage, carrots, cauliflower, eggplant, garlic, green beans, kale, leeks, onions, peas, peppers (all kinds), potatoes (sweet and white), spinach, sprouts (all kinds), squash (all kinds), string beans, and tomatoes are especially recommended for their nutritional value. One extra beneficial factor could be added by buying organically grown vegetables.

Foods to Skip

An anti-ageing diet plan has no place for foods like red meat, poultry, fish, milk, cheese, and eggs. Thousands of studies indict these foods for their role in the current epidemic of heart disease, cancer, and other degenerative conditions. For longevity, and youthful life, you will have to avoid all animal foods.

Similarly, refined carbohydrates such as white sugar, white flour, and processed foods are also a taboo for those following the anti-ageing diet. Refined carbohydrates have had their vitamins, minerals, and fibre stripped away, so they're of little nutritional value.

In contrast, complex carbohydrates are good because they retain their nutrients and they're converted to blood sugar more slowly. This prevents fluctuations in your blood sugar level, reduces fat storage, and supports weight loss and maintenance. As a bonus, when you eat a lot of complex carbohydrates, your diet automatically becomes low in fat and protein. In fact, because the foods have such good nutritional profiles, you can eat as much as you like.

An Anti-ageing Secret

Slowing down the process of ageing is possible. The body is designed to heal and repair itself with the aid of proper nutrition. The body requires two vital materials to complete this - energy and raw material. These two requirements are needed to maintain the cell's proper functions. The body is made up of cells and all cells are living. All living things need food. Each cell needs the proper food to keep it strong. Cells die and replace themselves at various intervals. To understand anti-ageing, understand that when a cell replaces itself it has three options that it can replace itself with:

1. A cell may replace itself with a weaker cell each time. A cell will do this if it hasn't had the right nutritional foods available to it. This process is called degeneration.
2. A cell can replace itself with the same strength cell. This means the body doesn't improve. That is, you have a chronic condition.
3. The cell is capable of replacing itself with a stronger and better cell. This will happen only if the cell has an abundance of energy and the right raw materials. This process is called regeneration. Regeneration is an anti-ageing process.

Many of the foods that we have been told are good for us in actual fact may cause degeneration. Foods which usually cause degeneration and ageing are high levels of carbohydrate, sugar, milk (especially homogenized milk), tea, coffee, chocolate, cola, cigarettes, white flour, microwaved food, chemicals such as fluoride, artificial sweeteners, alcohol, processed foods, colourings, additives, monosodium glutamate, preserved meat, margarine, vegetable oil, canola oil, olestra, hydrogenated oils, deep fried foods, chips, puffed grains, soy products which have not been fermented (soy milk and tofu) and meat and eggs raised by 'normal' methods which have many toxins and hormones.

Foods which can help regeneration and anti-ageing include fruit and vegetables especially sprouts, green leafy vegetables, legumes (such as lentils), Celtic sea salt, spirulina, seaweed, wheat grass juice, barley greens, Aloe Vera, antioxidants (e.g. vitamin C, vitamin E, Pycnogenol, coenzyme Q10), olive oil, evening primrose oil, foods with omega 3 fatty acids (flaxseed oil) and omega 4 and 5 fatty acids (evening primrose and fish oil).

In addition, frequent drinks of pure water are crucial. Health problems and the anti-ageing process would improve if we would just drink more water.

Nutritionists like to divide food into a number of different groups. I suggest that you think about dividing food into two groups. One group produces acids when it is digested. The other group produces alkalis when it is digested. Our bodies are constantly producing waste products, like the exhaust gases coming from the back of your car. Waste products are acidic. They are called toxins. Toxins cause tiredness, pain and ageing. Therefore, if you want more energy and less pain and anti-ageing, you need to eat less acid-producing food.

Foods that produce acids are carbohydrates and proteins. 'Foods' such as tea, coffee, soft drinks, sugar, flavourings, artificial sweetener and preserved meats are even more acidic i.e. toxic. And pollutants (like heavy metals) and pesticides are even worse.

To neutralise an acid you need an alkali. The only foods that produce alkalis are fruit and vegetables, particularly leafy, green vegetables, such as sprouts, parsley and cabbage. That is why people should eat lots of fruit and especially vegetables, for an anti-ageing effect. We all know that raw is best, when it comes to vegetables. And steamed is much, much better than boiled (as it retains the vitamins and minerals), and boiled is a hundred times better than fried.

Once you begin to understand this, it is easy to see why so many people are suffering from health problems. Have a look at what people put into their shopping carts, the next time you are at the supermarket. You will find a whole lot of white bread, soft drinks and preserved foods. And have a look at what people have on their plate next time you are in a restaurant. Lots of carbohydrate and protein, and very few vegetables, except maybe for salad.

This is not to say that we don't need protein and complex carbohydrates. We do. The key is balance. We need to balance the acid-producing foods we eat with much more alkali-producing foods, especially if we suffer from symptoms such as tiredness, pain, illness, gas and skin problems.

The other thing to bear in mind is that the body has hundreds of different chemical reactions going on, for which it needs at least 90 different things, including vitamins, minerals and essential fatty acids. Therefore, people need more variety in their diet to ensure that they get everything their body needs, for effective anti-ageing.

The anti-ageing diet includes a minimum of eight fruits and vegetables, lots of fibre-rich whole grains and legumes, non-fat milk products, and other natural foods. The anti-ageing activity plan includes both weight lifting and some type of aerobic activity, like walking, running, bicycling, or swimming.

There are some supplements you can add to this diet and exercise program that might give you an added boost, but only if you are eating and moving well.

Vitamin Supplements

What are the supplements that might help turn back the hands of time?

Vitamin E should be top on your list of supplements to consider. Not only are there hundreds of studies showing this vitamin lowers heart-disease risk, but recent evidence suggests it also might help protect your memory. The brain is exposed to a hefty dose each day of oxygen fragments called free radicals that damage the membranes and components of brain cells, possibly contributing to memory loss as we age. People who consume hefty doses of anti-free radicals or antioxidants also show the least memory loss and the best concentration as they age. Even animals fed diets fortified with vitamin E learn faster and remember more. Limited evidence suggests that vitamin E also might slow the progression of Alzheimer's disease.

How Much should you Take?

You can get some vitamin E from nuts, seeds, and oils, but not enough to prevent ageing. A safe supplemental dose is between 100 IU and 400 IU. Natural vitamin E is more potent than synthetic vitamin E.

Besides vitamin E, what other Supplements are Worth Considering?

Calcium. I know you've heard it before, but people still need to be reminded to boost their calcium intakes to lower their risk for not only osteoporosis, but possibly colon cancer and hypertension, and pre-eclampsia in pregnancy.

If you don't drink at least three glasses of non-fat milk or cups of yoghurt, or drink calcium-fortified soymilk or orange juice, then you need to take a calcium supplement. Since most people get at least 600mg from their diets, you really only need to fill in the gaps by taking about 500mg from a supplement.

Which Ones are Best?

Either calcium carbonate or calcium citrate supplies the most calcium per pill. You also need vitamin D, so make sure your multi-vitamin contains 200 IU to 400 IU of this vitamin, which is essential for calcium absorption and getting the calcium into bones.

Caution About Excess Intake

There are some people who believe that good eating can be avoided just by popping some vitamin supplements. This can't be further from the truth. Vitamin pills cannot compensate the nutritive value of a balanced diet. There are some vitamins that can have harmful effects, when consumed in excess.

Vitamin A – It is fat-soluble and the excess of this vitamin can be stored in the liver or other fatty tissues. An overdose can led to toxic effects and problems like insomnia, dry and flaky skin and headaches.

Vitamin Bs – The best way of taking the vitamins in this category is through vitamin B-complex capsules but vitamin B6, if taken in large doses (more than 50 mg a day), over a long period of time can cause nerve damage.

Vitamin C – Excessive intake of vitamin C can aggravate kidney stones because it increases the secretion of oxalic acid and uric acid.

Vitamin D – The best source of this vitamin is natural sunlight. An excess intake of this vitamin in any other form can lead to symptoms like drowsiness, constipation and loss of appetite. Too much of it, over a long period of time, can also cause damage to the kidneys.

Vitamin E – Too much of this vitamin can cause minor stomach upsets, but for those taking tablets to thin the blood, it can cause excessive bleeding. Those who are taking anti-coagulants to treat thrombosis should not take this vitamin unless the dosage is recommended by their doctor.

This should work as a warning to those who believe that vitamin supplements can only cause good health and nothing else. It is best to get the required dosage of vitamins through a healthy and balanced diet rather than rely on vitamin pills.

Fish Oils

For millions of years, our ancestors ate diets rich in a type of fat called omega-3 fatty acids, the fats once found in wild game and now found primarily in fish oils. Estimates are that our ancestors consumed an average of up to 10 grams a day, while today we consume less than one gram daily. While saturated fats in meat and dairy products are storage-type fats, fish oils are structural fats that are important components of cell membranes and hormone-like compounds in the body that possibly protect against a host of ills, from heart disease and cancer to even memory loss and depression. Even babies need these fats to ensure normal brain and vision development.

Although an optimal daily dose has not been identified, general consensus is at least two to three servings of fatty fish per week (salmon, mackerel, herring). Also, heart attack risk might decrease by 50 percent when people consume daily at least 200mg of the omega-3 fatty acids in supplements or in foods.

The 12 Top Anti-Ageing Foods

Many of what are considered signs of ageing—wrinkled skin, a fading memory, diminished physical capacity and an increased susceptibility to infection—are actually little more than deficiencies of critical chemicals called antioxidants. You don't have to sit by and watch your body disintegrate. Instead, you can eat the following foods to help hang on to and replenish your bio-mechanical vitality. Just about any fruit or vegetable will make contributions to your quest for youth; here are 12 you shouldn't ignore.

Avocado

True, avocado is high in fat, but much of it is "good" fat, the mono-unsaturated type, which resists oxidation. Avocado is high in glutathione, an antioxidant which helps neutralize fat in other foods. Research also suggests that eating avocado lowers and improves cholesterol better than a low-fat diet does.

Berries

Blueberries have more antioxidants called anthocyanins than any other food—in fact, 3 times more than the second-richest sources, red wine and green tea. Both blueberries and cranberries help ward off urinary tract infections. And a study showed that older people who ate strawberries had the lowest rates of all kinds of cancer.

Broccoli

The green stuff provides an awesome array of antioxidants. Scientists at John Hopkins Institute discovered a particularly strong one called sulforaphane. Served to animals, the broccoli chemical stoked the activity of detoxification enzymes that slashed cancer rates by two-thirds. Broccoli is packed with vitamin C, beta-carotene, indole, glutathione and lutein, and is also a rich source of the trace metal chromium, which is a life extender and protects against the ravages of out-of-control insulin and blood sugar.

Cabbage

People who ate cabbage once a week compared with once a month had only 66 percent of risk for colon cancer, one study found. Cabbage also seems to deter stomach cancer. Savoy cabbage (the crinkly type) is the strongest one; you can eat it raw or lightly cooked, for the best effect. The betacarotene, 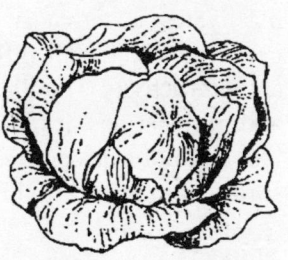 indoles, glucoinolates and isothiocyanates in these vegetables may prevent certain cancers.

Carrots

These are legendary in fighting off ageing diseases. In a recent study, men eating a couple of carrots a day lowered blood cholesterol by 10 percent. Many studies pinpoint beta-carotene, carrots' main antioxidant asset, as a powerhouse against ageing and disease. People with low levels of beta-carotene in their blood are more apt to have heart attacks, strokes and various cancers.

Citrus Fruit

The National Cancer Institute has called the orange the "complete package of every class of natural anticancer inhibitor known, including carotenoids, terpenes, flavenoids and vitamin

C". Grapefruit, too, has a unique type of fibre that reduces cholesterol dramatically and may reverse the ageing disease atherosclerosis.

Grapes

Grapes contain 20 known antioxidants that work together to fend off oxygen free-radical attacks that promote disease and ageing, according to researchers at the University of California. The antioxidants are in the skin and the seeds, and the more colourful the skin, the greater the antioxidant punch.

Onions and Garlic

They might give you bad breath, but they help prevent cancer, thin your blood (discouraging clots) and raise the good type (HDL) of cholesterol. Red and yellow onions (sorry, not the white ones) are the richest of all foods in quercetin, a celebrated antioxidant that inactivates cancer-causing agents, inhibits enzymes that spur cancer growth and has anti-inflammatory, antibacterial, anti-fungal and antiviral activity. The allicin in garlic lowers the bad LDL cholesterol and triglycerides. It reduces blood pressure, boosts immunity and has antibiotic properties. Allium compounds are also found in spring onions, leeks, chives and shallots.

Spinach

Heavy in lutein, an anti-ageing agent which rivals beta-carotene for effectiveness, spinach also has beta-carotene plus a good dose of folic acid, a brain and artery protector.

Tomatoes

These are the richest source of lycopene, which new research suggests helps to preserve mental and physical functioning among the elderly. High levels of lycopene also reduce your risk of pancreatic cancer.

Green Tea

Research indicates that green tea may have some anti-cancer effect. It contains polyphenols, a kind of antioxidant. Green tea has also shown promising results for heart and liver diseases.

Oats

An excellent heart medicine. About half cup of dry oat bran or a cup of dry oatmeal puts a dent in your blood cholesterol and regulates the sugar level.

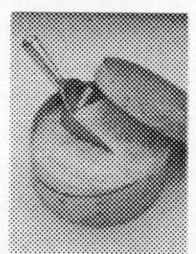

Want to Remain Young?

Who doesn't? Here are some sure shot tips to keep you looking at least ten years younger than your age. A word of caution – don't expect miracles or overnight results, patience and discipline in following these rules will get you to the ultimate goal.

- Drink a glass of vegetable juice every day. Raw vegetable juice is full of known and unknown antioxidants, which in turn help in reducing free radical activity.
- Eat at least 5 servings of fruits and vegetables every day. The goodness of fruits and vegetables can never be undermined.
- Consume less oil. Excessive fat intake increases free radical activity. The excess fat that we consume in the form of oily snacks gets oxidised and rancid thereby producing a burst of free radical activity in the body. These free radicals are in excess of what the body can normally diffuse and cause ageing. Recycling the used oil is another harmful habit practised by most homemakers. It is a dangerous practise, to say the least.
- There are endless brands of tea in the market but making a choice for a better one can work wonders. Have you ever wondered how the Japanese retained their youthful looks? Well, the answer is quite simple - they drink green tea and eat a lots of fish. If you want similar benefits, switch to green tea as it has lot of antioxidants.
- Avoid sugar and refined flour for the same reason.
- Stop smoking. Smoking can age people by ten years apart from playing havoc with their health. It ages the skin and brings on wrinkles around the mouth and eyes.
- Eat up to ¾ of your capacity. This helps your digestive machinery to work better.

Include at least two calcium rich foods every day. It could be a bowl of low fat curd and some soya bean or bowl of rajma, chowli or channa. Curd helps increase the friendly bacteria in your gastro-intestine tract and also looks after your bone health. Soya bean, apart from helping you maintain healthy bones, has innumerable health benefits.

- Exercise or take a brisk walk for 30-40 minutes regularly for at least 6 days a week.
- Stay involved with family and friends. Being loved and a sense of belonging work as shock absorbers and help rev up immunity.
- Maintain a positive outlook.
- Do what really makes you happy. Apart from this, doing meaningful work with honesty and living one's life in a conscientious, responsible way all contribute to inner peace and longevity.

■ ■

7. The Yin And Yang of Food

Yin, Yang and Diet

In traditional oriental medicine practice, diet is an integral part of the treatment. Shiatsu practitioners often recommend a change in the diet plan for their patients. According to them, various types of foods differ in their physical, mental, spiritual and emotional effects. This energy is split into two parts known as Yin and Yang. Yin is where energy is expanding and yang is where it is contracting. Food can be divided into three main types–those that are 'balanced', and some that are yin and some that are yang.

Yin Foods:

MILK

Alcohol	Honey
Sugar	Oil
Fruit juices	Spices
Stimulants	Most drugs (such as aspirin)
Tropical vegetables and fruits	Refined foods
Most food additives of a chemical nature	

Yang Foods:

POULTRY

Seafood	Eggs
Meat	Salt
Fish	Cheese

Balanced Foods:

SEEDS

Nuts	Vegetables

Cereal grains   Beans
Sea vegetables
Temperate fruits (such as apples and pears)

The balance between yin and yang is very important to the body. For example, it plays a major role in the production of hormones such as progesterone, glycogen and insulin and the expansion and contraction of the lungs. A balanced way of eating, mainly from grains, beans, seeds, nuts and vegetables, is important as this will help achieve the energy balance in the meridians, organs and chakras. When these two opposing forces of yin and yang are in harmony and balanced, physical and mental health is bound to result.

Food For All Seasons

Almost all scriptures and ancient medical texts mention the potency of certain foods during specific seasons. Nature has created vegetables and fruits according to the requirements of the season. If watermelons and cucumbers are generally found during the summers, there is a reason for it. These vegetables and fruits have a high water content and quench thirst and that is the reason they are available during the hot months, whereas fruits and vegetables like peas, cabbage, cauliflowers and apples are available during the winter time because they have certain warming properties in them. The human body responds differently to different seasons. Just as our bodies need a different type of clothing in different seasons, we also need to eat differently. It is advisable to eat the right kind of food during the appropriate season because of the natural goodness that is contained in them.

Just as our body requires more energy to cater for the normalising of body temperature during winters, it needs a lot of moisture during the summer to combat the drying and dehydrating effect of high temperature. Food is, therefore, to be planned to provide the required contents.

Winter Food

Apart from having a physical nature to it – like proteins, fats, carbohydrates – food also has a thermal nature. It has warming and cooling properties e.g. ginger, garlic, most grains like wheat, *jowar, bajri*, onions, *sarson,* green chillies, pepper, mustard have a warming effect on the body. Dates, honey and jaggery are sweeteners that have a warming effect. All animal products are essentially warming.

During winter, our food should be geared to cater for the increased energy required to combat the coldness in the atmosphere. Since it takes a lot of energy to keep the body at the normal temperature during the winter, our food should be such that it gives our body warmth and the energy that is necessary to maintain peak performance. Foods have specific properties. Some foods help increase energy, others calm the mind, some foods reduce mucous, some provide warmth and others cool the body.

Indian households consume more of the whole grain products and pulses during the winters. Pulses like *kabuli chana, rajma,* black *dal* are consumed in substantial quantities and so are the stuffed 'parathas' made out of cauliflower, peas and radish etc. There is strong logic in this – these pulses are difficult to digest during the hot months but they provide the warmth essential to our bodies during the winter months. Cooking methods that require longer cooking time impart more warming qualities to food e.g. cooking vegetables on slow fire, imparts more warming qualities than stir frying. Moderately cooked food, especially in winter is better digested; its nutrients are better assimilated, which in turn give warmth and energy to the body.

Makkai ki roti and *sarson ka saag* is popular not because of its taste alone but because it contains the essentials required to provide warmth and energy to the body. Whole grains like *makka, jowar, bajra* etc. are also wholesome food which should be consumed in large quantities during winter.

Dry fruits have a strong position in the menu during winter because of their warming properties. They provide the body with essential oils and energy besides warmth. Hot soups with spices like pepper, ginger, garlic and onions are also a popular food item during the cold season and those who eat non-vegetarian foods can increase intake of eggs, fish, and chicken to at least 3-4 times a week. Alcohol also has a warming effect on the body. For those of you who take alcohol, red wine should be a good choice. It has many health benefits. A glass of wine a day can help you make severe winters more bearable.

Summer Food

Just as the body needs more energy to combat the winters, it needs less supply of energy during the summer time. It is the season for light food and lots of fluids. This is the season when ice-cold fresh lime juice is more popular than coffee and tea, unless it is the cold coffee or lemon tea. This is also the time of the year for salads and cold soups like the Russian salad and the *gazpacho*.

'Cool as a cucumber' is a saying that is as old as the language. Cucumbers are known to have a cooling effect on the body and provide the much-needed water content to keep the normal hydration balance in the body. Melons, gourds, mango and lemons are available in plenty. These have high water content and are cooling in nature.

Summer food should contain the least oil and fat, as the body already excretes a lot of sweat and grime. Pulses, which are lighter in nature, like *moong* or *masoor* should be eaten while the heavier ones should be avoided. Whole grains like *makkai* and *bajra* are definitely to be avoided and so should whole pulses like *rajma* and *chana*, simply because they are difficult to digest.

Although most people do not like gourds like the bottle gourd, ridge gourd, snake gourd etc, they are very high in moisture content and very cooling in nature. That is the reason that nature has provided them to help us tide over the harsh months of summer.

Radish has a cooling thermal nature. In summers some people suffer from nosebleeds and headaches or body rashes. In such conditions, radish juice is very useful as it helps in detoxification and cleansing of the body toxins.

The intake of cool drinks like coconut water, buttermilk and lime juice needs to be increased, while caffeine containing beverages like coffee and tea should be minimised.

Monsoon Food

Monsoon months are notorious for water contamination and spread of digestive disorders including diseases such as jaundice and typhoid. Salads, which contain raw vegetables, are one of the likeliest sources of contamination. It is, therefore, essential that vegetables be washed and cleaned well before being used.

Avoid raw vegetables as the water may be contaminated and cause diarrhoea.

Hot and energising soups can be quite an invigorating experience during the rainy season. This is also the time when vegetables, which are not very high in water content can be eaten without worry. Indian monsoons are the transitory phase between summer and winter and almost all vegetables and fruits that belong to both the summer and winter season are also available during monsoon.

Foods to be Avoided

Meats	Canned, salted or smoked meat, fish, bacon, cold cuts, chipped or corned beef, frankfurters, ham, sausage, frozen fish fillets, clams, lobsters, crabs, oysters, scallops, and shrimp
Cereals	Quick cooking cereals, enriched cereals containing sodium compounds.
Breads and starches	Regular breads, hot breads and pastries prepared with baking soda or regular baking powder, cakes and mixes.
Vegetables	Frozen green peas and lima beans.
Fruits and juices	Crystallised or glazed fruit, dried or frozen fruit with sodium sulphite or sodium benzoate added and regular tomato juice.
Fats	Salted butter or margarine, bacon, olives, salted nuts, commercial mayonnaise, peanut better and cheese, French dressings etc.
Milk	Powdered, condensed, milk.
Beverages	Instant cocoa mixes.
Sweets	Brown sugar, molasses, commercial syrups, candies, jams, and jellies containing sodium preservatives.
Desserts	Baking mixes, commercial ice-creams etc.
Miscellaneous	Mustard, pickles, chilli sauce, meat sauces, relishes, soy sauce, and monosodium glutamate.

Persons with severe cardiac conditions should avoid the following gas forming foods – broccoli, cauliflower, cabbage, Brussels sprouts, Cole slaw, green peppers, onions, corn, cucumbers, radishes, turnips, sweet potatoes, melon, raw apples and lima beans. Avoid stimulating beverages like strong coffee and strong tea.

Special Diets

People suffering from various ailments are advised to cut out certain items or include some items in their food. Here are some items be avoided by people who are on the low-triglyceride and low-cholesterol diets.

Low Triglyceride Diet

Foods not allowed

Sugar	Sherbet	Alcohol	Caviar
Candy	Fruit ice	Chocolate	Cake
Pie	Coconut	Liver	Jam
Pastry	Coconut oil	Sweet breads	Jelly
Doughnut	Lard	Brains	Syrup
Honey	Condensed milk	Butter	Kidney
Cocoa butter	Marmalade	Cram	Fried food
Sausage	Molasses	Sour cream	Potato chips
Soft drinks	Mayonnaise	Pork	All foods containing sugar

Low Cholesterol Diet

Foods not allowed

Chocolate	Coconut	Coconut oil	Cocoa butter	Sour cream
Lard	Butter	Mayonnaise	Palm oil	Salted pork
Frankfurters	Sausage	Kidney	Liver	Brain
Sweet bread	Lobsters	Shrimp	Clams	Crabs
Cheeses	Fried foods	Potato chips	Fritters	Doughnuts
Pancakes	Pastry	Cookies	Cake	Whole milk
Evaporated milk	Condensed milk	Avocado		

Foods that can Make Our Skin Glow

Slathering a whole lot of creams and lotions on the skin cannot make it glow. It is balanced and nutrient-rich diets that can bring a soft incandescence to the skin making it look beautiful. Vitamin A, C and E are increasingly important because of their antioxidant capabilities. Free radicals are thought to be the cause of many diseases from cancers to colds. The free radicals damage a person's DNA, causing unwanted changes in the basic building blocks of the cells. This damage can often be prevented, and sometimes be reversed, with the healing properties of antioxidants.

Vitamin A works as an antioxidant of invaluable worth. It disarms molecules called the free radicals. These are unleashed by white blood cells whenever the skin is irritated by sun, smoke or pollution. If left unchecked free radical molecules cause damage to healthy skin collagen, which brings firmness to the skin. Damaged collagen causes wrinkles, slacken the skin and can lead to skin cancer. Vitamin A is found in many yellow and green vegetables, egg yolk, butter, liver and fish oils. Retinoids, the active ingredients in vitamin A, can reduce and prevent wrinkles, brown spots etc and bring about improvement in skin texture and tone.

Beta-carotene contained in carrots, leafy vegetables, sweet potatoes, squash, cantaloupes, meat, butter and cheese, also contains agents that act as free radical scavengers and protect the body cells. A combination of vitamin A and beta-carotene can work wonders in protecting the skin from harmful effects of free radicals.

Vitamin C or ascorbic acid is found in vegetables and citrus fruits. It acts as an antioxidant by scavenging and quenching free radicals throughout the body. The harmful effects caused by sunlight's UVA and UVB rays can be nullified by vitamin C and this can control skin damage.

Vitamin E like vitamin A and C, is an antioxidant. When combined with Vitamin C, it acts as a powerful protective factor against the UVB rays of the sun. Vitamin E is present in vegetables, oils, seeds, corn, soy, whole-wheat flour, margarine, nuts and some meats and dairy products. Vitamin E is also used on the skin for protection against sunburn.

To find the required amount of antioxidants, it is necessary to eat a varied diet.

Quick Energy Foods

It's only 3 p.m. but your mind is wandering and your productivity has come to a grinding halt. You wonder how you are going to get through the rest of the day. You are not an exception, there are many people who find their energy level ebbing by mid-day. The reason for this drained-out feeling is a wrong mix of foods.

Eating right can boost energy levels and keep us at our peak level through the day. Food is body fuel and adding high-energy choices to the diet can keep the engine running at peak performance.

One of the most common problems seen in the lack-energy crowd is that they hardly take any breakfast. Lack of breakfast is one of the biggest energy-sappers known. Apart from that, we need to constantly refuel our body with a meal or snack every five to six hours. Some of the right kinds of energy packed foods taken at right intervals can keep the energy levels on a constant high.

If you're like most people, that means it's time to reach for a cup of coffee or a candy bar to give you some extra boost before quitting time. But quick-fix solutions such as caffeine and sugar ultimately deplete your energy rather than enhance it; the former can leave you feeling jittery (and interfere with needed sleep later on), while the latter can lead to a post-sugar-high crash.

Here's what you can do:

Stock up on Carbohydrates

Fibre-rich complex carbohydrate foods are a fantastic source of energy. Unlike fats and proteins, carbohydrates are stockpiled in the muscles and liver as glycogen, a readily available energy source that our bodies can tap whenever required. These fuel reserves ensure that the energy levels stay at an even keel.

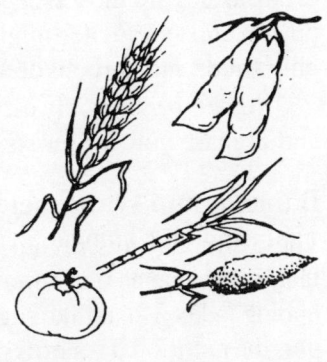

The best fuel for muscles is carbohydrate—either simple sugars (such as naturally occurring sugars in fruits and juices) or complex carbohydrates (the starches in whole grain products, rice, cereal, oatmeal and other plant foods). These carbohydrates provide not only energy but also important vitamins and minerals.

You store only carbohydrates—not protein or fats – in your muscles in the form of sugar called glycogen. During hard exercise, you burn this glycogen for energy. When you deplete your glycogen stores, as can happen during repeated days of hard training and a low carbohydrate diet, you feel exhausted. Eating high carbohydrate foods (cereal, pancakes, bread, fruit, vegetables, potato, pasta) on a daily basis can help you cope better with the energy requirements, especially if you are on the high activity daily schedule.

Eating lots of sweets and sugary foods for "quick energy" before you exercise may hurt your performance. Here's why: After you eat any kind of concentrated sugar (soft drinks, candy, donuts, etc.) your body secretes insulin, a hormone that carries sugar from your blood into the muscles. Exercise, like insulin, also helps carry sugar into the muscles. The combined effect of insulin with exercise can cause your blood sugar to drop abnormally low. You may experience hypoglycaemia (low blood sugar) and feel light, shaky, tired and uncoordinated. If you are hungry, droopy and craving a quick energy boost prior to exercise, you don't have to eat sugar for energy. A simple snack of crackers, fruit or bread can perk you up!

You should eat carbohydrate-rich foods and fluids within 1 to 2 hours after hard exercise to replace the glycogen that you burned off. Muscles are most receptive to refuelling at this time. A simple post-exercise refueller might be fruit juice — a rich source of not only fluids and carbohydrates but also potassium and vitamins.

Remember that only carbohydrates quickly refuel your muscles and prepare you for bursts of quick energy.

Bananas and Watermelon

These simple fruits rev up energy as fast as sugary sweets do. In fact, ripe bananas rate almost as high as table sugar on the energy-upping index. But unlike sugar, fresh fruit gives you a stamina boost plus the nutritional benefits of fibre, vitamins and minerals. Bananas also contain lots of potassium, an electrolyte that helps maintain normal muscle and nerve functions. Unlike some nutrients, potassium isn't stored by the body for long periods, so your potassium level can drop during strenuous exercise due to excessive sweating. The results of low potassium level in the body are irregular heartbeat, slower reflexes and a feeling of confusion apart from aching muscles.

An added bonus is that there's no food quite as portable as a banana. Since watermelon can be a bit messy to eat at your desk, cut some into chunks the night before and stash in a plastic container. (Dates, mangoes, papaya and pineapple also rank high on the energy-revving scale.)

Carrots and Potatoes

Just like sugary snacks and soft drinks, carrots and potatoes can up your blood sugar to an all-time high. In fact, mashed and baked potatoes are on a par with pure honey when it comes to how quickly they're digested and absorbed into your bloodstream. But unlike junk food, these good-for-you eats supply a host of important nutrients (such as vitamins A and C, folic acid and potassium) along with that energy blast. Keep a bag of baby carrots in your desk drawer and you'll be less likely to make an afternoon trip to the canteen.

Cornflakes and Shredded Wheat

Even without added sugar, wholesome cereals such as corn flakes, instant oatmeal, puffed rice and shredded wheat top the list of breakfast foods that provide quick energy. These morning eats tend to be digested slowly, which means that blood sugar levels stay stable. Adding skim milk and fruit to the mix helps produce a slow but steady release of glucose into the bloodstream to fuel your muscles and brain throughout the day.

Oats is another wonder food which has a rich blend of fibre, which means your body gets a steady stream of energy as the carbohydrate flows slowly into your bloodstream. A porridge made of oats is likely to keep you on a 'high' for a long time.

Fish

This is a reputed brain booster. High protein fish like tuna, seerfish, mackerel, sardines or pomfrets contain an amino acid called tyrosine. Tryrosine, when digested, helps manufacture the brain 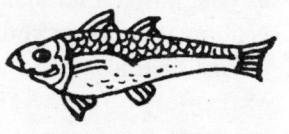 chemicals called norepinephrine and dopamine which are natural brain 'uppers' and bring your brain to high alertness. If you want to wake up for that crucial meeting, just try a sandwich with some tuna slices thrown in!

Water

If you're not drinking at least eight cups of water a day, especially in warm weather or if you work out regularly, you're setting yourself up for dehydration and lagging energy. Don't wait until you feel parched to fill your glass: At that point, your body is already suffering. Make a habit of setting a full glass of water on your desk all day long.

Five Foods for Better Health

Want to look great and live longer? The secret isn't a new miracle drug or surgical technique. It's not even a new exercise program (though exercise couldn't hurt). No, the real secret can be found in the foods you eat. Here are five foods that will help prevent disease and make us look and feel great.

Soy

A fantastic food for our health. It lowers cholesterol, and it reduces the incidence of osteoporosis as well as breast cancer and heart disease. Staving off osteoporosis is of particular importance because so many women are at risk for it. Soy is not just tofu; you can find it in soy nuts, which are a great snack food and good for sprinkling on a salad, or soy burgers.

Salad

Certain salad ingredients are going to do more for your body than others. For example, using leafy greens (such as spinach) as your base rather than lettuce is going to increase your intake of folic acid. Folic acid is extremely important for pregnant women and women 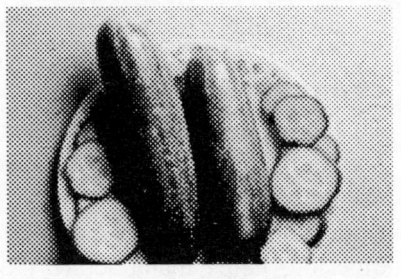 in their childbearing years. If you include carrots in that salad, you're getting a powerful antioxidant that reduces the risk of heart disease and cancer. Broccoli should also make an appearance. It is a great source of calcium as well as vitamin C. Of course, it's not a salad without tomato, and in tomatoes you'll find another powerful antioxidant that reduces the risk of prostate cancer. It becomes more potent, however, when it is consumed in the form of cooked tomato products, such as stewed tomatoes or fresh tomato sauce.

Fish

This is rich in omega-3 fatty acids, which are extremely good for the body. They decrease the incidence of heart disease and breast cancer. When selecting a fresh piece of fish at the market, you want to look for a firm fillet that has a healthy sheen to it and that doesn't smell "fishy". Fish is very easy to prepare. The best way to maintain the omega-3 fatty acids is to poach the fish. Season it with a little bit of parsley and some freshly ground pepper, maybe a little bit of coarse salt; you'll need only about one minute per inch of thickness for cooking time. Very easy, very tasty and great for you!

Bread

Whole grains provide us with fibre, and fibre has been shown again and again to reduce the risk of colon cancer. Aim for at least 30 grams of fibre per day. Take care, however, to consume brown bread rather than white.

Blueberries

They are practically a dessert item, so it's fun to be able to include them as part of a healthy diet. And it's easy to convince the kids to eat them as well. Much like cranberries, they are used to reduce the incidence of urinary tract infections. Blueberries are also a powerful antioxidant, reducing the risk of many cancers as well as things such as memory loss.

Five Energy-Draining Habits

You drink lots of water. You exercise regularly. You even take multivitamins. So what is it that's robbing the spring from your step?

Skimping on the Necessities

Lack of sleep, exercise and good nutrition are the biggest energy-drainers in most people's lives.

Eating Meat, Poultry and Eggs

They're all rich in the amino acid tryptophan, which helps induce sleep. So go light on these eats early in the day.

Gulping Caffeine

Coffee, tea and diet colas are stimulating, but they don't provide carbohydrate calories, which are the source of true energy. If you rely on caffeine for energy, you'll soon find yourself running on empty fuel tank.

Snacking on Sugary Treats

Sugar gives you instant energy that fades super-fast.

Gorging on Big Meals

You'll exhaust yourself trying to digest all that food. Instead, eat small amounts of food more often.

Are you guilty of the above energy-draining habits? Counteract that behaviour by consuming plenty of your body's favourite fuel - carbohydrates. But how you eat them is just as important as what you eat. For instance, if your goal is to maintain your blood sugar levels and avoid a late-afternoon slump, your best bet is to consume small meals every three or four hours that contain at least 50% carbohydrates. And since different foods are absorbed into your body at different rates, eating a nutritious combination of foods at every sitting-such as a serving of low-fat yoghurt, a cup of fruit salad and an *idli* or a *chapati* or a slice of brown bread for breakfast-ensures that you'll get an instant boost of energy, plus enough fuel to sustain you throughout the day.

Fruitful Facts

Nature has given us a bountiful of gifts, in the form of fruits and vegetables. Each fruit comes with its own, unique medicinal properties, which are vital to the normal functioning and growth of the body. These elixirs from nature contain a treasure of minerals, vitamins, salts, acids and easily digestible sugars. They are nature's own tonics, and medicines, dispensed in the most delicious manner.

Fruits and vegetables should form three-fourths of our diet to keep us free from disease and ensure good development of mind, body and emotions.

Fruits should never be peeled, cooked or preserved. They are best taken in the raw form. In fact, for best value, they should not be taken in the juice form. When juiced, the fibre-benefits are lost and when cooked, they lose a large part of their energy-providing sugars, carbohydrates and nutritive salts. Here are some gems from the fruit basket.

Apples

Apples are rich in iron and contain a big amount of pectin, which is so valuable in healing and curing all kinds of intestinal disturbances. They help in lubricating and stimulating the peristalsis, and keep the bowel movements in an excellent condition. This valuable fruit is excellent for a sluggish liver because it steps up the flow of bile and increases active elimination from the system.

For people suffering from gout and rheumatism, they are invaluable because of the rich phosphorus content. Apples are also helpful in alleviating complaints like calculus and stones and acid formations due to the high malic acid content, which neutralises sedimentation. Apples are known to be blood purifiers, body cleansers and bowel regulators apart from being invaluable in cosmetic uses.

Amla

It is probably the richest natural source of vitamin C, which is assimilated easily by the human system and is useful in curing haemorrhage, diarrhoea, and dysentery. It has a high nutritional and medicinal value. In the ayurvedic system of medicine, it is used to cure several kinds of ailments. It is also an effective laxative.

Amla is helpful in alleviating acute bacillary dysentery, constipation, and biliousness.

Banana

A popular and easily available fruit, it is also highly affordable and contains a lot of nutrients. The thick outer covering of this fruit is anti-bacterial and anti-contaminative. Its alkaline ash content corrects the acid balance and helps in curing problems like constipation and colonic instability.

Bananas are rich in minerals like calcium, magnesium, phosphorus, iron, copper and mineral salts. This fruit is known as a complete food because of its vitamin A, B, C and D content. The high carbohydrate content (22%) in bananas can only be matched by grapes. Due to its nutritive value it is known as an excellent body-builder and is recommended for sportsmen, athletes and those involved in hard, manual labour.

Since bananas act as a non-irritant food, they are also given to people who need bland diets or are suffering from ailments such as typhoid, gastritis, fever, peritonitis, etc.

Surprisingly, it is a fruit that is given for weight gain as well as weight loss, for diarrhoea as well as constipation. Banana is the only fruit that can be taken by patients of chronic ulcers.

Fig

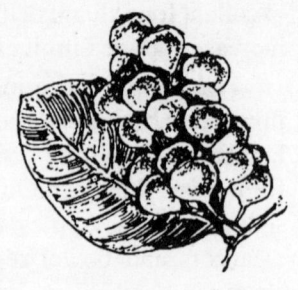

Figs are highly nutritive in their natural as well as dried forms. Being rich in almost all necessary nutrients in digestible form, figs are known to be great health promoters and are recommended for growing children. Dry figs have a high content of sugar. This fruit is generally used for most digestive problems and for constipation.

Currants

They contain sugar and malic acid. These are berries containing 85-90% water and just about 8-12% fruit sugar with very little protein and pectin, just like all other kinds of berries. Currants are especially useful for sore throats and colds.

The Invaluable Berries

Berries

Berries also contain malic acid apart from 10-16% sugar and some minerals. These are alkaline in nature and stimulate bile flow thus creating a beneficial effect on kidneys and bowels.

Raspberries

These contain almost all essential elements required for the body e.g. potassium, magnesium, sulphur, calcium, phosphorus, chlorine and iron. Raspberries have a high vitamin B and C content, too.

Blackberries

They contain copper, sugar and iron and provide quick regeneration of blood and are good for digestion. They find use in the treatment of diarrhoea, fever and kidney disorders.

Blueberries

They are a good source of copper and iron as well as a natural insulin-like chemical called myrtillin. They are useful in alleviating constipation and help the pancreas in maintaining normal blood sugar levels.

Grapes

They contain proteins, carbohydrates, vitamin A and B, minerals like potassium, iron, calcium, manganese, chlorine, fluorine, sulphur and phosphorus. The iron that is present in organic form is easily assimilated so it is invaluable for the anaemic. This fruit is a storehouse of sugar, potassium and vitamins, which aid nutrition. Grapes are also considered laxatives because of their tartaric acid content. They also stimulate the liver and kidneys besides eliminating toxins from the system.

The alkaline nature of this fruit helps in general cleansing and blood purification. It is also helpful in detoxifying the system. An exclusive diet of grapes is recommended to counteract cancerous growths. Grapes are an excellent tonic, which revitalise the body and repair tissue waste.

Mango

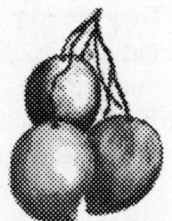

Mangoes provide wholesome nourishment to the body because they are rich in sugar, vitamins A, and C. mangoes are known to be good laxatives and diuretics.

Papaya

It is a delicious fruit with invaluable medicinal properties. It is one of the most alkaline foods which helps in maintaining the body's alkaline balance. It also contains vitamin A, B ad C as well as traces of vitamin D. It is rich in calcium, phosphorus and iron. The digestive enzymes papain contained in the fruit make it invaluable for people suffering from constipation, digestive disorders, and kidney stones. The enzymes papain and papyatin help in digesting the protein in acid, alkaline or neutral medium.

Orange

Oranges are known for their protective effects against various diseases. Rich in vitamins B, C and calcium, they are very healthful and provide quick energy to the body. Oranges are useful in maintaining the digestive organs, kidneys, blood vessels and nervous system. They also prevent gingivitis and pyorrhoea and strengthen the teeth.

The high content of minerals like lime and magnesium, bone building elements, make it very valuable for growth of children. The potash contained in its juice is alkaline in reaction. Because of its quick absorption and utilisation, orange juice is preferred as nutrition during convalescing. The fibre in this fruit acts as a digestive tract cleanser.

Peach

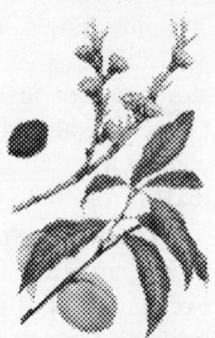

Peaches have a high water content of about 80%. They neutralise the acidity in blood because of their mineral and vitamin content. Peaches are excellent laxatives.

Grapefruit

Grapefruits contain more citric acid than oranges but less of sugar. They are low in carbohydrates and proteins but rich in fruit acids and salts, potassium and vitamins A and B. This fruit contains chlorine and sulphur, which makes it an excellent cleansing agent of the stomach and its mucous lining. Grapefruit stimulates appetite and helps in digestion by increasing the flow of digestive juices. It is also a natural antiseptic.

For people suffering from arthritis and rheumatism, it brings relief as it acts as a solvent of the chalky deposits in the joints and muscles. For diabetics it is a good fruit because it prevents diabetic gangrene due to the vitamin C content in it. Grapefruit is also recommended as a restorative during fever.

Pomegranate

Pomegranates are rich in sugar and citric acid. They are also a rich source of iron. This fruit is good in alleviating problems like diarrhoea.

Lemon

Lemons are loaded with citric acid, alkaline minerals and vitamin C. It improves the liver functions by increasing the flow of bile. It is also rich in calcium and the acid contained in it helps in curing digestive problems. The high percentage of citric acid makes lemon an invaluable medicine in many ailments. It also contains potash and vitamin B. A very effective cure for rheumatism, gout and arthritis, lemons help in dissolving the uric acid. It finds use in curing catarrh, sore throat, cough and diphtheria, also.

Pineapple

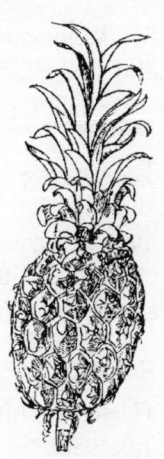

It contains an active digestive enzyme known as bromalin, which is a digestant. The fruit helps in the digestion of animal and vegetable protein. It is invaluable as a digestive agent in cases of acidosis and in dyspepsia. Pineapple raises the alkaline content of the blood and helps in getting rid of excess water in cases of oedema. In bronchitis, pineapple juice has been found to be an excellent medicine in softening the mucus. It is also used as a laxative.

Dry Fruits

These are a valuable part of the diet because they are rich in concentration of essential minerals including iron. They also contain potassium, a mineral needed for healthy nerve function, heart beat regulation and lower blood pressure. Dried fruit also contain magnesium, an important bone mineral and essential for release of energy in cells.

The sweetness of dried fruit comes from natural sugar, or fructose. The fructose contained in dried fruit doesn't cause the blood sugar levels to fluctuate as rapidly as the sucrose and glucose used in confectionary. So, dried fruit is an ideal substitute for chocolates and other sugary snacks. Diabetics can also take dried fruits in controlled amounts because fructose doesn't require the action of insulin to be metabolised by the body.

Dried fruit contain lots of fibre. Dried apples, figs and apricots are among the best sources of fibre, both soluble and insoluble. The rich combination of nutrients makes dried fruits a valuable snack. When there is no time for a proper meal, dried fruits can be taken without any problems because they keep the energy levels from dipping too low and help replace any essential mineral lost through perspiration.

Dried fruit helps in relieving premenstrual syndrome and help keep symptoms like depression, headaches and cravings in check. The magnesium levels, one of the causes of premenstrual syndrome, can be maintained by eating dried fruit during the time of a period. The potassium content in dried fruit, especially banana, may help minimise the premenstrual bloating due to water retention.

When soaked in water overnight, dried fruits like figs, raisins and prunes, can act as an effective remedy for constipation.

Dates

They are a valuable source of wholesome nutrition, easily assimilated and digested. They contain a very high percentage of sugar in the natural form. Being rich in protein, lime, iron, vitamins and other essential food constituents that are a wholesome substitute of cane sugar, they form a nutritious food.

Raisins

These are high in alkaline content because of which they are invaluable in curing acidosis. They are also quick energy food.

Apricots

Apricots are rich in iron and minerals, they are good body cleansers and good for toxaemia and constipation.

Food for Vitality and Vigour

Have you noticed how the youth of modern times lack the vim and vigour that our forefathers had at young age? The food we eat doesn't contain the same nutritional value it did earlier. Today our soils are also depleted of essential nutrients? One example: you would have to eat 75 bowls of spinach today to get the same iron content in one bowl of spinach just 50 years ago!

Even if we don't eat processed foods there isn't enough nutrition in food. We need to supplement! Living in a fast-paced society, we eat food too fast. How many people do you know who chew each mouthful of food for one full minute?

Chewing your food sends signals to the brain telling it how much digestive fluids are needed to digest the food that is going into the stomach. For example, if you eat a large pizza and chew and gulp it down only enough to tell the brain there was just a little of it, then the body doesn't have enough digestive fluids to break down the food enough to get nutritional value from it. Also, chewing signals the brain as to what kind of digestive juices are needed in the stomach. For example: When you eat protein your body produces an acid to break it down; when you eat starch your body produces an alkali.

Optimum Nutrition for Vigour and Vitality

Everyone eats in order to remain active but how many of us really believe in eating healthy and nutritious food? Do we eat to perform at the peak of our capacity or maintain vigour and vitality?

Diet plays a vital role in the maintenance of good health and in the prevention and cure of disease. In the words of Sir Robert McCarrison, one of the best-known nutritionists, "The right kind of food is the most important single factor in the promotion of health; and the wrong kind of food is the most important single factor in the promotion of disease."

Human body is made up of millions of cells, and tissues which need different kinds of nutrients to maintain themselves and regenerate continuously. The different glands and organs need vital nutrients for peak performance. For all bodily functions like metabolic, hormonal, mental, physical or chemical, the body requires specific nutrients. Foods that provide these nutrients are thus one of the most essential factors in building and maintaining health.

Lack of nutrition often leads to lowered resistance in the body and results in the failure of the body to fight off diseases. There is an elaborate healing mechanism within the body but it can perform its function only if it is abundantly supplied with all the essential nutritional factors.

It is believed that human cells need at least 45 chemical components and elements. Each of these 45 substances, called essential nutrients, must be present in adequate amounts. The list includes oxygen and water. The other 43 essential nutrients are classified into five main groups, namely carbohydrates, fats, proteins, minerals and vitamins. All 45 of these nutrients are vitally important and they work together. The lack of any of these vital elements can result in disease and ill health.

These nutritional deficiencies occur on account of various factors, including the intense processing and refining of foods, the time lag between harvesting and consumption of vegetables and fruits, the chemicals used in bleaching, flavouring, colouring and preserving foods and the chemical fertilisers, fungicides, insecticides and sprays used for treating the soil.

Research has also shown that diseases produced by combinations of deficiencies can be corrected when all the nutrients are supplied, provided irreparable damage has not been done. A well-balanced and correct diet is thus of utmost importance for the maintenance of good health and the healing of diseases. Such a diet obviously should be made up of foods that in combination would supply all the essential nutrients. A diet that contains liberal quantities of

a. seeds, nuts, and grains,
b. vegetables and
c. fruits will provide adequate amounts of all the essential nutrients. These foods have, therefore, been aptly called basic food groups and a diet containing these food groups is an optimum diet for vigour and vitality.

Seeds, Nuts and Grains

These are the most important and the most potent of all foods. Grains like millet, wheat, oats, barley, brown rice, beans and peas are all highly valuable in building health. Wheat, mung beans, alfalfa seeds and soya beans make excellent sprouts. Sunflower seeds, pumpkin seeds, almonds, peanuts and soya beans contain complete proteins of high biological value.

Seeds, nuts and grains are also excellent natural sources of essential unsaturated fatty acids necessary for health. They are also good sources of lecithin and most of the B vitamins. They are the best natural sources of vitamin C, which is perhaps the most important vitamin for the preservation of health and prevention of premature ageing. Besides, they are rich sources of minerals and supply necessary bulk in the diet. They also contain auxones, the natural substance that plays an important role in the rejuvenation of cells and prevention of premature ageing.

Vegetables

As stressed earlier, vegetables are an extremely rich source of minerals, enzymes and vitamins. Faulty cooking and prolonged careless storage, however, destroy these valuable nutrients. Most of the vegetables are, therefore, best consumed in their natural raw state in the form of salads.

There are different kinds of vegetables. They may be edible roots, stems, leaves, fruits and seeds. Each group contributes to the diet in its own way. Fleshy roots have energy value and good sources of vitamin B. Seeds are relatively high in carbohydrates and proteins and yellow ones are rich in vitamin A. Leaves, stems and fruits are excellent sources of minerals, vitamins, water and roughage.

To prevent loss of nutrients in vegetables, it would be advisable to steam or boil vegetables in their juices on a slow fire and the water or cooking liquid should not be drained off. No vegetable should be peeled unless it is so old that the peel is tough and unpalatable. In most root vegetables, the largest amount of mineral is directly under the skin and these are lost if vegetables are peeled. Soaking of vegetables should also be avoided if taste and nutritive value are to be preserved.

Fruits

Like vegetables, fruits are an excellent source of minerals, vitamins and enzymes. They are easily digested and exercise a cleansing effect on the blood and digestive tract. They contain high alkaline properties, a high percentage of water and a low percentage of proteins and fats. Their organic acid and high sugar content have immediate refreshing effects. Apart from seasonable fresh fruits, dry fruits, such as raisins, prunes and figs are also beneficial.

Fruits are at their best when eaten in the raw and ripe states. In cooking, they loose portions of the nutrient salts and carbohydrates. They are most beneficial when taken as a separate meal by themselves, preferably for breakfast in the morning. If it becomes necessary to take fruits with regular food, they should form a larger proportion of the meals. For the maintenance of good health, at least one reasonably large serving of uncooked fruits should form part of the daily diet. In case of sickness, it will be advisable to take fruits in the form of juices.

Milk-Oils-Honey

The three basic health-building foods mentioned above should be supplemented with certain special foods such as milk, vegetable oils and honey. Milk is an excellent food. It is considered as " Nature's most nearly perfect food." The best way to take milk is in its soured form - that is, yoghurt and cottage cheese. Soured milk is superior to sweet milk as it is in a pre-digested form and more easily assimilated. Milk helps maintain healthy intestinal flora and prevents intestinal putrefaction and constipation.

High quality unrefined oils should be added to the diet. They are rich in unsaturated fatty acids, vitamin C and F and lecithin. The average daily amount should not exceed two tablespoons. Honey too is an ideal food. It helps increase calcium retention in the system, prevents nutritional anaemia besides being beneficial in kidney and liver disorders, colds, poor circulation and complexion problems. It is one of the nature's finest energy-giving foods.

A diet of the three basic food groups, supplemented with the special foods, mentioned above, will ensure a complete and adequate supply of all the vital nutrients needed for health, vitality and prevention of diseases. It is not necessary to include animal protein like egg, fish or meat in this basic diet, as animal protein, especially meat, always has a detrimental effect on the healing process. A high animal protein is harmful to health and may cause many of our common ailments.

A Healthy Menu

Based on what has been stated above, the daily menu of a health-building and vitalising diet should be on the following lines:

First Thing in the Morning

A glass of lukewarm water mixed with the juice of half a lemon and a teaspoon of honey, or a glass of freshly squeezed juice of any available seasonable fruit such as apple, pineapple, orange, sweet lime and grapes.

Breakfast

Fresh fruits such as apple, orange, banana, grapes, or any available seasonal fruits, a cup of buttermilk or unpasteurised milk and a handful of raw nuts or a couple of tablespoons of sunflower and pumpkin seeds.

Mid-morning Snack

One apple or a banana or any other fruit.

Lunch

A bowl of freshly prepared steamed vegetables using salt, vegetable oil and butter for seasoning, one or two slices of whole grain bread or chapattis and a glass of buttermilk.

Mid-afternoon

A glass of fresh fruit or vegetable juice or any available fruit.

Dinner

A large bowl of fresh salad made up of green vegetables, such as tomatoes, carrot, cabbage, cucumber, red beet and onion with lime juice dressing; any available sprouts such as alfalfa seeds, and mung beans; a warm vegetable course, if desired; one tablespoon of fresh butter, cottage cheese or a glass of buttermilk.

One can alter the basic elements with an eye to individual needs and taste. Care should be taken, however, to include food items from each group. If you prefer certain kinds of grains, you could substitute those for the ones given above. For instance, those who like vegetable soups before their main course, could easily include them in their meals, for added beneficial effect. In certain parts of the country buttermilk is generally served with the meal, which again is a very desirable inclusion.

The TCM Way to Increase Vitality and Vigour

Do you experience low energy after eating certain foods? Have you wondered why when you've hardly eaten any calories you still have a hard time losing weight and eventually just keep gaining?

Traditional Chinese Medicine has a unique way of looking at food. Besides the known macro and micro-nutrients (carbohydrates, proteins, vitamins and minerals, etc.), they go by the seasonal growth, colour, textures and flavours of food. Whole foods have a stimulatory effect on innate organic functions. Being 4000 years old, TCM is a highly effective form of medicine practiced throughout the world. It not only includes acupuncture, herbology, moxibustion (heat therapy) and Qi Gong (exercise therapy), But also food therapy as one of its primary modalities!

In the old days in China, the acupuncturist's (TCM practitioner's) job was to keep their patients well. If their patients fell sick they didn't get paid, so education and participation in all aspects of their patients' health was of utmost importance, and food was and still is right at the top of the list.

We require our bodies to endure high emotional and physical stress as some of us work 50, 60, 70 hours a week without vital nutritional support. So how long do we logically think we can keep going before things begin to break down? Even by our thirties, many of us have found that we've worked hard getting through college, pursued a career, perhaps bought a house, but we've done it all on half a tank—and poor fuel at that. Now when it's time to enjoy our success, we find ourselves with debilitating health problems that may have been easily prevented with a little time and care.

People have lost their sense of eating in harmony with the seasons. Before refrigeration most of our food was eaten seasonally, now we don't even know what that means. Ancient sages of all lands, meticulously studied nature, and its effect on our health. As a result, their entire system is about living in harmony with nature, through which their bodies would be healthy.

The Five Elements

The Chinese envisioned five elements in nature with each element corresponding to the each of the different seasons. Besides this, they assigned specific foods, flavours, activities, emotions, colours, sounds, etc. These elements are Wood, Fire, Earth, Metal and Water.

Wood

The wood element corresponds to spring. Its corresponding flavour is sour. This corresponds to the need, especially in spring, for an increase of vitamin C (which as ascorbic acid is sour tasting). It is at this time that we should especially forage for the early spring greens and vitamin rich edible weeds. These foods tend to eliminate the build-up of higher levels of mucus necessary for bodily warmth during the winter season.

Fire

The summer element is fire. Its flavour is bitter. Some greens have a bitter flavour like dandelion root and greens, some salad greens. Therefore raw foods such as these are only supposed to be eaten in season, otherwise they cause an imbalance. While during the summer it is appropriate to eat more raw foods, people with allergies should limit the intake of cold raw food, because they need

160

internal warmth and have to increase their body's immunity to antigens. This is shocking to most people because our understanding of nutrition is that fruit and salads are always good. This is not true with the energetic dietary principles of traditional medicine.

Earth

The earth represents the period between summer and winter, the mid-season and its flavour is sweet. This is not the kind of strong sweet most of us consider. Rather it is the need for full sweet which includes whole protein and complex carbohydrates such as beans, whole grains, root vegetables, winter squash, animal protein, etc. These foods are nutritionally dense and all bodily tissues. Carbohydrates are necessary for energy, while protein is used to heal and repair the cells of the body as they naturally break down and helps us maintain metabolic strength.

Metal

This corresponds to autumn or fall. The flavour is spicy (acrid or pungent) and includes garlic, onion, ginger and mint. This flavour disperses congestion, and stagnation, increases blood and lymph flow while counteracting mucous production. These foods are especially important to help prevent colds and flus that typically occur during the fall and winter seasons.

Water

This represents winter, and its flavour is salt. This is a full or wholesome salt, naturally found in nature and rich in an abundance of vital trace minerals. Refined kitchen salt is refined to be pure sodium chloride with none of the accompanying buffering minerals. Good quality mineral-rich salt is important to maintain the proper ratio of potassium in the blood and cells.

It is through the chemical reaction of potassium and sodium, called electrolyte balance, that nutrients and waste is carried to and from the cells. Because salt tends to retain fluid in the body, it is important to maintain pliability and softness of the various tissues and organs of the body. Certainly in winter, a time of storage, we may need more salt to help us retain body fluid and other nutrients. Over millennia, the ancient Chinese discovered how these flavours harmonized with the organs, either toning up or sedating them according to our individual requirements and the seasons. The teachings of Taoist priests always included knowledge of therapeutic diet.

What does this mean to those of us who upon catching a cold, believe that the best foods are fruit juices such as sugar-rich orange juice because of its purported high vitamin C content? Though the vitamin C is good, the cold temperature and nature of the juice is definitely wrong. The concept of cold essentially means to lower our body metabolism, while heat means to raise it. Therefore, when we consume cold natured foods out of season it throws the chemistry of our blood and body out of balance with the seasons and climatic environment. As a result, our immune system and digestion become weaker and we are more prone to external diseases such as colds and flus.

The same is true for people who are overweight. They can deprive themselves of necessary calories and eat cold natured foods such as yoghurt, fruit, salad, etc. And because they have depressed or cooled down their metabolism, once they start eating normal food, they gain all the weight with a vengeance.

The Chinese think of the stomach (called the "spleen" in TCM) as a cooking receptacle that likes to be about 100 degrees Fahrenheit. Of course, this heat, besides actual temperature, is biochemical and consists of hydrochloric acid and the various digestive enzymes that are used to break down food. We could consider this like our internal fire metabolism. The therapeutic objective is to harmonize the individual with the season, innate constitution, lifestyle and activity so that the body is better able to maintain itself. Breath, food and proper rest are primary to health. The job of the spleen, in TCM physiology, is to transform food into blood and ultimately the very substance of the body itself.

The spleen, therefore, represents the innate warmth and strength of our metabolism and, as per Chinese teachings, it doesn't like to be cold and damp because these are the two energies that will lower overall physical metabolism. The results are symptoms of coldness and dampness including weak digestion, abnormal weight gain, lowered immune system, etc. Too much cold or raw foods weaken our digestive and assimilative capacity on all levels and it is much like placing a cold, wet log into a burning fireplace. This creates smoke. In the body's metaphorical sense, 'smoke' is expressed as gas, bloating and heaviness. In general, decreased assimilation of important nutrients including vitamins and minerals eventually leads to chronic disease. This is why all traditional healing systems stress the importance of maintaining good digestion.

The Dietary Principles of Traditional Medicine, Including TCM, are:

- Eat whole natural unprocessed food.
- Consume more high quality nutrient dense foods that are rich in vitamins and minerals. This includes good quality protein found in fish and range fed poultry and other animals as well as light vegetable sources of protein such as soy products and various beans.
- Be sure to include various seaweeds for important trace minerals and organic vegetables of all kinds. Also include one or two servings of whole grains such as brown rice once or twice a day. Again, the use of grains may need to be modified according to individual requirements.
- Try to avoid refined foods, foods with artificial colouring and preservatives, coffee and other stimulants, alcohol, drugs including marijuana. Limit dairy products and all foods with saturated fats and oils. Primarily use olive and sesame oil for cooking and dressings.
- Have three good meals a day with breakfast or lunch being the largest and the evening meal the lightest. Many do better, and even lose weight, on a schedule of having six light and balanced meals during the day.
- Balanced means a proper ration of protein and carbohydrate at each meal. Eat foods, as they are seasonally available in your climatic environment. Foods that are imported from warmer climates tend to alter the chemistry of our blood to acclimatize us to the foreign environment.
- Learn to acknowledge and accept your unique constitutional requirements based on ancestral history and innate constitutional type.
- Take time to focus on your food when you eat. Fully experience its colours, flavours and textures, which are an

expression of their energies. Take time to carefully chew each mouthful, since digestion begins in the mouth.

- Avoid overconsumption of cold or raw foods unless it is in the warmer seasons. When you are tempted by sugary foods and foods that lack wholesome, balanced qualities, let this be a sign that you need to eat more balanced, protein-rich foods first. Quite often, our abnormal and addictive cravings will automatically vanish if we follow this principle.

- Avoid excess. Learn to eat everything in moderation. While it is not good to waste food, we live in a society of repletion so that learning to leave a little food in the plate each time we eat ultimately makes good soil compost.

Aphrodisiac Foods

Love potions have been described since the fourth century B.C. Today there are thousands of foods thought to have aphrodisiac properties.

Theophrastus (4th century B.C.), a Greek botanist, recommended a love potion that included a leafy plant called mandrake soaked in vinegar. Supposedly, mandrake contains substances that create the sensation of "feeling high". According to ancient Indian recipes, love can be enhanced with a mixture of black pepper, honey, chilli peppers, and mandrake. Apicius, who lived during the reign of Julius Caesar and authored the first known cookbook, suggests a stew of onions, pine kernels, and various herbs as an effective love potion.

Today there are thousands of foods presumed to have aphrodisiac properties. These include (raw) seafood, chocolate, wine, spices, and even sugar. An Italian psychiatrist, Willy Pasini, has actually researched foods that supposedly have romantic properties. Dr. Pasini discovered during animal experiments that maize, a type of corn, contains a compound called "tryptophan" that combines with other chemicals in the brain to act as an aphrodisiac.

To intensify passion, Dr. Passini also recommends that you add sparkling wine, fruit, and chocolate to your meals. However, Dr. Passini is not the first to promote fruit as an aphrodisiac. Apricots and peaches are considered erotic symbols by the Chinese. Ancient Greeks celebrated each new crop of figs, while ancient Jews considered fruit an important part of the mating ritual.

According to the *Cambridge World History of Food:* "Aphrodisiacs were first sought out as a remedy for various sexual anxieties including fears of inadequate performance as well as a need to increase fertility. Procreation was an important moral and religious issue and aphrodisiacs were sought to insure both male and female potency."

Can food really be an aphrodisiac? Yes, indeed! Just read what *Encyclopaedia Britannica* has to say on this subject:

"...the psycho-physiological reaction that a well-prepared meal can have upon the human organism. The combination of various sensuous reactions - the visual satisfaction of the sight of appetizing food, the olfactory stimulation of their pleasing smells and the tactile gratification afforded the oral mechanism by rich, savoury dishes - tend to bring on a state of general euphoria conducive to sexual expression."

All cultures have foods that are considered aphrodisiac. Each culture has a different item of food that it considers as a panacea for sexual inadequacies. For example, saffron in Spain, bird's nest soup in China, camel's hump among the Arabs, cocoa for the Aztecs, are popular as potent cures for impotency. It was said, for example, that Montezuma had 600 concubines, and to satisfy them he drank 50 cups of cocoa per day from a golden goblet. Over time, almost every interesting or exotic foodstuff, particularly if reminiscent of the male or female sex organs, has been used to inspire desire and stimulate performance: bananas, peaches, berries, figs, dates, asparagus, nuts, seeds, stuffed dates, sea urchins, to name a few.

Why Certain Foods?

In ancient times a distinction was made between substances that increased fertility versus ones that simply increased sex drive. One of the key issues in early times was nutrition. Food was not so readily available as it is today.

Under-nourishment creates a loss of libido as well as reduces fertility rates. Substances that "by nature" represent "seed or semen" such as bulbs, eggs, snails were considered inherently to enhance sexual powers. Other types of foods were considered stimulating by their "physical resemblance to genitalia".

It's important to realize these food substances were documented by ancient Greeks like Pliny and Dioscordes in the first century AD and later by Paul of Aegina (seventh century). Later more credence was given to foods that "satisfied dietary gratification".

Other foods deemed to have these aphrodisiac qualities were derived from mythology. Aphrodite, the love goddess, was said to consider "sparrows" sacred because of their "amorous nature" and for that reason they were included in various aphrodisiac brews.

There was not always agreement upon what foods were actually aphrodisiacs or "anaphrodisiacs" (decreasing potency). The ancient list included Anise, basil, carrot, salvia, gladiolus root, orchid bulbs, pistachio nuts, rocket (arugula), sage, sea fennel, turnips, skink flesh (a type of lizard) and river snails.

The ancients suggested you steer clear of dill, lentil, lettuce, watercress, rue, and water lily.

Some Popular Aphrodisiacs

Aniseed

A very popular aphrodisiac with many culinary uses. It has been used as an aphrodisiac since the Greeks and the Romans, who believed the herb had special powers. Sucking on the seeds is said to increase desire.

Asparagus

It could be due to its phallic shape that the asparagus is regarded as an aphrodisiac.

Almond

A symbol of fertility throughout the ages. The aroma is thought to induce passion in a female. There is an ancient practice of serving Marzipan (almond paste) in the shape of fruits for a special after-dinner treat.

Arugula

Arugula or "rocket" seed has been documented as an aphrodisiac since the first century A.D. This ingredient was added to grated orchid bulbs and parsnips and also combined with pine nuts and pistachios. Arugula greens are frequently used in salads and pasta.

Avocado

The Aztecs called the avocado tree *Ahuacuatl* which translated means "testicle tree". The ancients thought the fruit hanging in pairs on the tree resembled the male testicles.

Bananas

The phallic shape of this fruit is partially responsible for the popularity of the banana as an aphrodisiac. An Islamic tale recounts that after Adam and Eve succumbed to the apple they started covering their nudity with banana leaves rather than the fig. From a more practical standpoint, bananas are rich in potassium and B vitamins, necessities for sex hormone production.

Basil *(sweet basil)*

It is said to stimulate the sex drive and boost fertility. Also said to produce a general sense of well being for body and mind.

Chocolate

The Aztecs referred to chocolate as "nourishment of the Gods". Chocolate contains chemicals thought to effect neurotransmitters in the brain and a substance related to caffeine called *theobromine*. Chocolate contains more antioxidant (cancer preventing enzymes) than does red wine.

Carrots

It is believed to be a stimulant for males. The phallus-shaped carrot has been associated with stimulation since ancient times and was used by early Middle Eastern royalty to aid seduction.

Coffee

Caffeine is a well-know stimulant but remember, too much and it becomes a depressant.

Coriander *(cilantro seed)*

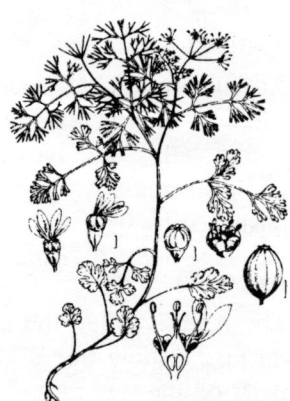

The Arabian Nights tells a tale of a merchant who had been childless for 40 years, but was cured by a concoction that included coriander. The book is over 1,000 years old so the history of coriander as an aphrodisiac dates back far into history. Cilantro was also used as an appetite stimulant.

Figs

An open fig is thought to resemble the female sex organ and is traditionally considered a sex stimulant.

Garlic

The 'heat' in garlic is said to stir sexual desires. Garlic has been used for centuries to cure everything from the common cold to heart ailments.

Ginger

Root raw, cooked or crystallized, ginger is a stimulant to the circulatory system.

Honey

Many medicines in Egyptian times were based on honey including cures for sterility and impotence. Medieval seducers plied their partners with Mead, a fermented drink made from honey. Lovers on their honeymoon drank mead and it was thought to "sweeten" the marriage.

Liquorice *(licorice)*

The Chinese have used licorice for medicinal purposes since ancient times. Chewing on bits of licorice root is said to enhance love and lust.

Mustard

Believed to stimulate the sexual glands and increase desire.

Nutmeg

It was highly prized by Chinese women as an aphrodisiac. In large quantities nutmeg can produce a hallucinogenic effect.

Oysters

They were documented as an aphrodisiac by the Romans in the second century A.D as mentioned in a satire by Juvenal. He described the wanton ways of women after ingesting wine and eating "giant oysters". In reality, oysters are very nutritious and high in protein. Their zinc content makes them scientifically aphrodisiacal.

Pine Nuts

Zinc is a key mineral necessary to maintain male potency and pine nuts are rich in zinc. Pine nuts have been used to stimulate the libido as far back as medieval times.

Pineapple

Rich in vitamin C, it is used in the homeopathic treatment for impotence.

Shiitake Mushroom

Shiitake (she-e-ta-kay) mushroom is a non-pathogenic fungus that can be grown on low valued oak logs. Shiitake cultivation began in Japan centuries ago. Japan accounts for approximately 80 percent of the total production of the mushroom.

Also called lentinus edodes, it is the most popular edible mushroom in Japan. It has been the foundation of traditional medicine in Asia for thousands of years. It is reputed to be a tonic, a stimulant, an aphrodisiac, and an aid in the prevention of cerebral haemorrhagic strokes.

Truffles

The Greeks and the Romans considered the rare Truffle to be an aphrodisiac. The musky scent is said to stimulate and sensitise the skin to touch.

The Scientific Explanation

As mentioned above, zinc is one of the major nutrients necessary for boosting sexual drive; it is found in red meat, oysters, pumpkin seeds, organ meats, and organic eggs. Refined sugar, flour and rice are zinc deficient. Deficiency causes whitening of the hair and nails, loss of hair, poor circulation, impotence, lack of ovulation or menstruation, psychotic symptoms, slow wound healing, and hyperactivity in children. Whole grains, while they contain zinc, also contain phytates, which inhibit its absorption; soaking the grain overnight before cooking inactivates the phytates. According to experts, the other nutrients required for sexual potency are:

Potassium (all fruits and vegetables),

Selenium (organic butter, herring, tuna, whole wheat, Brazil nuts, and sesame seeds),

Manganese (nuts, seeds, and whole grains),

Phosphorus (abundant in whole grains, pumpkin and sunflower seeds, and brewers' yeast),

Vitamin E (eggs, whole grains, organ meats, sweet potatoes, almonds, and leafy green vegetables),

Vitamin C (all fruits and vegetables, especially citrus, cantaloupe, strawberries, broccoli, tomatoes, and parsley),

Vitamin A (liver, eggs, sweet potatoes, carrots, fish liver oil), B complex vitamins (abundant in whole grains, brewer's yeast, and liver).

The inability to reach orgasm in both men and women is linked with a lack of histamines. Histamine production appears to be triggered by folic acid, vitamins B6 and B12. Foods rich in folic acid include organ meats, asparagus, leafy greens, peanuts, mushrooms, whole grain cereals, lean beef, egg yolk—all of which have been considered aphrodisiac.

Foods that Dampen Desire

Sexual energy wanes with malnutrition, lack of protein, fat or calories. Sugar, alcohol, and caffeine, especially when used to excess, can interfere with the absorption of the nutrients mentioned above and result in impaired sexual function. A high-sugar vegetarian diet, as well as an over-reliance on soy foods may both dampen desire.

Certain traditions that favour celibacy stress foods known to reduce the interest in sex - in Japan, for example, tofu is considered "cooling" to the sex organs and therefore favoured in monastic vegetarian diets. Unfermented soy foods like tofu and soymilk may block zinc absorption because of their phytate content whereas miso and shoyu don't do that. Other "cooling" foods are cucumber, turnips, kale, and cabbage. All these foods contain anti-thyroid factors, not favourable for a healthy sex life, because the thyroid regulates sexual activity, desire, and fertility. These foods are best used moderately and together with other more energizing foods.

Truth and Myth

Of the various foods to which aphrodisiac powers are traditionally attributed, fish, vegetables, and spices have been the most popular throughout history. In none of these foods, however, have any chemical agents been identified that could effect a direct physiological reaction upon the genitourinary tract, and it must be concluded that the reputation of various supposedly erotic foods is based not upon fact but folklore.

Folklore had specified certain food elements as aphrodisiacs, based on their shape rather than therapeutic effects. So if an object resembled the genitalia, it possessed, it was reasoned, sexual powers; thus the legendary aphrodisiac powers of ginseng root and powdered rhinoceros horn. With the exception of certain drugs such as alcohol or marijuana, which may lead to sexual excitement by removing inhibitions, modern medical science recognizes a very limited number of aphrodisiacs.

So if you are prone to visiting a quack in the shady clinic located in a dubious area downtown for a quick cure to your problems in potency and sexual inadequacies, you are not likely to find scientific backing to many of the cures that he prescribes as aphrodisiacs. For a scientific approach, consult your physician.

■ ■

Table - 1: Calories Burnt in Various Activities (per minute)

Activity	Cal. expenditure per min.
1. Laying still	1.0
2. Sitting, standing, reading, writing, eating, playing cards and handsewing etc.	1.5
3. Driving car, tailoring	2.0
4. Washing floors, sweeping and ironing	2.2
5. Golf	2.5
6. Walking 5 km. per hour speed	3.0
7. Walking 7 km. per hour speed	4.5
8. Walking 9 km. per hour speed	9.0
9. Gardening, Weeding etc.	5.0
10. Cycling (depending upon speed)	3.5 to 8.0
11. Boxing, Rowing	12.0
12. Dancing	5.0
13. Table Tennis	5.50
14. Tennis	6.0
15. Swimming 3 km per hour speed	9.0
16. Football	8.0
17. Running (depending upon speed)	10 to 25
18. Other Exercises a) Light	2.5
b) Moderate	4.0
c) Severe	8.0

Table - 2: Daily Calories Requirement

Age	Calorie requirement per day
1. Upto 6 months	120 calories per kg. body weight
2. 7-12 months	100 " "
3. 1-3 years	1200 calories (for full body weight)
4. 4-6 years	1500 " "
5. 7-9 years	1800 " "
6. 10-12 years	2100 " "
7. 13-15 years (boys)	2500 " "
8. 13-15 years (girls)	2200 " "
9. 16-18 years (boys)	3000 " "
10. 16-18 years (girls)	2200 " "
11. Men	
a) Light work	2200 " "
b) Medium work	2800 " "
c) Heavy work	3400 " "
12. Women	
a) Light work	1900 " "
b) Medium work	2200 " "
c) Heavy work	2800 " "

Table - 3: Calorie Content of Common Food Items in Convenient Measures

A. Raw Foods

Item	Measure	Weight g.	Energy Cal.
Cereals			
Rice	1 Cup (small)	150	520
Wheat Flour	"	90	310
Millet Flour	"	90	300
Pulses			
Bengalgram	"	130	485
Other dals	"	135	460
Whole Pulses			
Greengram	"	140	470
Cowpea (lobia)	"	135	440
Rajmah	"	120	415
Soyabean	"	130	530
Green-leafy Vegetables	5 Bundles	100	62
Other Vegetables	–	100	105
Nuts and Oilseeds			
Almonds	10 no.	15	85
Cashewnuts	10 no.	15	95
Coconut (fresh)	1 no.	115	510
Coconut (dry)	1/2 no.	45	290

Item	Measure	Weight g.	Energy Cal.
Groundnuts	50 no.	15	85
Sesame seeds	1 tsp.	3	15
Oils/Vanaspati ghee	2 tsp.	10 ml.	100
Spices Chillie powder	1 tsp.	7	17
Coriander seeds	1 tsp.	7	20
Cumin seeds	1 tsp.	5	18
Fenugreek (Methi)	1 tsp.	6	20
Mustard seeds	1 tsp.	10	5
Garlic	7 pods	3	4
Onion	1 med.	50	30
Animal foods Egg (hen)	One	60	100
Mutton	–	100	194
Fish (lean)	–	100	100
Fish (fatty)	–	100	150

Notes: **tsp:** teaspoon (5 ml.), **tbsp:** table spoon (15 ml.),
1 cup (small) = 150 ml.

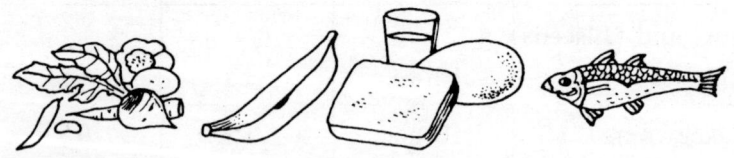

Table-3 (Contd.): B. Cooked Foods

Item	No. of Serving	Weight gms.	Energy cal.
Cereal preparations			
Rice	1 Cup	100	110
Idli "	60	75	
Plain dosa	"	40	125
Masala dosa	"	100	200
Phulka	"	35	80
Paratha	"	50	150
Upma	"	130	200
Sevian upma	"	80	130
Bread toasted	2 slices	50	170
Poha (Awal)	1 Cup	100	200
Dalia	"	140	165
Khichidi	"	100	210
Puri	1	25	80
Pulse preparations			
Plain dal	1 Cup	140	170
Sambhar	"	160	81
Chole/Sundal	"	150	115
Vegetable preparations			
With gravy	1 Cup	130	130
Dry	"	100	115
Bagara Baigan	"	170	230
Vegetable kofta	"	145	220
Fried snacks			
Bhaji	1	7	35
Samosa	1	65	210
Kachori	1	45	200
Potato Bonda	1	40	100
Sago vada	1	30	100
Masala vada	1	20	56

Item	No. of Serving	Weight gms.	Energy cal.
Vada	1	20	65
Dahi vada	1	80	170
Vegetable cutlet	1	30	70
Chutneys			
Coconut/ground nuts/til/coriander	1 tbsp	25	64
Tomato	1 tbsp	20	10
Non-Vegetarian preparations			
Boiled egg	1	50	86
Omlette	1	65	155
Fried egg	1	50	155
Mutton curry	1 cup	145	240
Chicken curry	"	125	260
Fish (fried)	2 pieces	85	220
Bakery products			
Biscuits	2	40	220
Cake	1	40	220
Vegetable puff	1	60	170
Pastry	1	50	350
Mathri	2	75	300
Sweets			
Laddu, burfi etc.	1	60	250
Halwa (Suji)	1 cup	130	430
Double ka meetha	"	105	280
Custard/puddings	"	110	180
Chikki	2	60	300
Jam/Jelly	1tsp.	7	20
Sugar	1 tbsp	15 ml.	20
Honey	1 tbsp	15 ml.	60
Jalebi	2 pieces	100 gm.	500
Gulab Jamun	”	50 gm.	400
Jaggery	1 tbsp.	15 gm.	56

Table-3 (Contd.): C. Salads

Item	No.	Weight gms.	Energy cal.
Beetroot	1	65	30
Cabbage	1	250	70
Carrot	1	40	20
Cucumber	1	90	12
Lettuce	6 bundles	100	20
Onion	1	50	25
Radish	1	60	10
Tomato	1	50	10
Turnip	1	100	30

D. Fruits

Item	No./ Quantity	Weight gms.	Energy cal.
Apple	1	100	65
Banana	1	80	90
Grapes	30	100	70
Guava	1	100	50
Jack fruit	4 pieces	100	90
Mango	1	250	180
Mosambi/orange	1	100	40
Papaya	1 piece	250	80
Pineapple	1 piece	100	50
Sapota	1	80	80
Custard apple	1	130	130
Watermelon/ Muskmelon	1 piece	100	15

E. Beverages

Item	Measure	Qty. ml.	Energy cal.
Coffee	1 cup	150	100
Tea	1 cup	150	60
Carbonated beverages	1 bottle	200	150
Fresh lime juice	1 glass	200	60
Squash	"	200	80
Syrups (sherbat)	"	200	200
Orange juice	"	200	150

F. Milk and Milk Products

Item	Measure	Weight gm./ Qty. ml.	Energy cal.
Milk (Buffalo)	1 cup	150 ml.	300
Milk (cow)	"	150 ml.	100
Curd (cow)	"	150 ml.	85
Butter milk (lassi)	"	150 ml.	45
Paneer	"	100 gm.	350
Ghee	2 tsp	10 ml.	100
Butter	3 tsp	15 ml.	100
Khoya (from whole milk)		100 gm.	400
Khoya (Butter separated)		100 gm.	200
Skimmed milk	1 cup	150 ml.	45
Cream	1 tbsp	15 ml.	50
Cheese	1 packet	30 gm.	100
Rabadi	1 cup	150 gm.	525

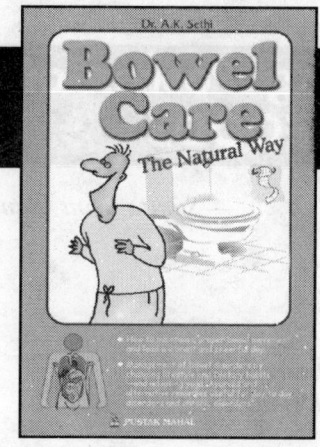

Bowel Care
The Natural Way

—*Dr. A.K. Sethi*

Good digestion is the key to a healthy body and sound mind. Considering today's eating habits, modern lifestyle and the stress and tension of hectic schedules, most of us suffer from digestive problems. In many cases, however, a person needs the right information and a little care in regulating his/her dietary habits and lifestyle.

Bowel Care is especially designed as an ideal self-help guide to all who suffer from such problems—or are likely to. Presented in an easy, lucid style with lively illustrations, it brings home to the reader a "Total Solution".

Written by a specialist in his field, it is a well-researched and simple work to provide relief to the readers.

The book highlights:

* ❖ Structure and functions of the Digestive System and related organs.
* ❖ Causes and symptoms of bowel disorders.
* ❖ Diagnosis and treatments of common digestive ailments.
* ❖ Management of bowel disorder through Diet, Yoga, Meditation and Ayurvedic treatments.

Demy Size • Pages: 112
Price: Rs. 60/- • Postage: Rs. 15/-

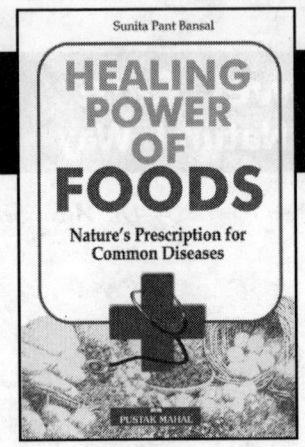

Healing Power of FOODS

—*Sunita Pant Bansal*

Nature's Prescription for Common Diseases

Hippocrates, the father of medicine, recognized that the medical therapy must be consistent with the nature and the design of the human body. He believed that the effective health care could not be separated from nutrition. He stressed prevention of disease by strongly recommending a balanced diet with a moderate and sensible lifestyle. Hippocrates wrote, "Natural forces within us are the true healers of disease... Everything in excess is opposed to nature... To do nothing is sometimes a good remedy." His philosophy was very much akin to the holistic health perspective of today.

The various foods provide not only nutrition to our body, but can prove to be medicinal too. 'Healing power of Foods' introduces all the main food groups to the reader, giving details about the medicinal uses of the commonly used foods from these groups. The tips given are simple, practical and effective. The healthy recipes at the end of the book complete the role of the various foods in providing nutritional as well as medicinal benefits.

Demy Size • Pages: 136
Price: Rs. 80/- • Postage: Rs. 15/-

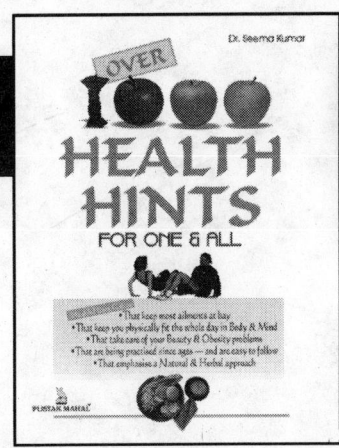

Over 1000 Health Hints
for one & all

—Dr. Seema Kumar

With ever-rising ground, water and atmospheric pollution, every other day, one hears the name of a new disease. Ever since, man began drifting away from Nature, he is falling into the trap of a materialistic lifestyle that has desensitised him. Today, we breathe air thick with exhaust fumes, eat processed junk food that has no nutritive value, drink toxic carbonated beverages and lead sedentary lives. All of this ensures that we are plagued with different kinds of problems at regular intervals.

This book shows you how to go back to Mother Nature to beat even the most troublesome and chronic ailments. With natural preventive measures that emphasise diet, exercise and herbal remedies, there are no fears of obnoxious side effects.

Whatever be your problem – diabetes, blood pressure, asthma, acne, menopause, obesity, stomach ailments, premature ageing or general complaints – this book shows you a safe, natural and enjoyable means to overcome it. Most of the ingredients mentioned in the book are the kind available in home gardens or off the kitchen shelf.

Once you have read this book from cover to cover, you need not rush to the doctor every now and then, but will be able to take care of your own and your family's health yourself.

Big Size • Pages: 168
Price: Rs. 80/- • Postage: Rs. 15/-